EXERCISE FOR PAIN RELIEF

THE HIDDEN TRUTH

MECHANISMS, STRATEGIES AND REMEDIES FOR PROFESSIONALS

DANIEL LAWRENCE

Copyright © 2023 by Daniel Lawrence

All rights reserved. No part of this publication may be reproduced, distributed or transmitted in any form or by any means, without prior written permission from the author. For information, contact the publisher Physio Books Ltd
(www.PhysioBooks.com).

The publisher has made every effort to acknowledge the original holders of any copyright material and to seek permission for use in this book. If this is not clear or if copyright holders have any queries, please contact the publisher so that a suitable acknowledgement can be agreed.

First published in 2023 by Physio Books Ltd, UK

Exercise for Pain Relief by Daniel Lawrence. 1st edn.

ISBN: 9798853477186

To Oliver and Lucas, my sons

ALWAYS STAY INQUISITIVE AND NEVER STOP LEARNING.

TABLE OF CONTENTS

PREFACE 6

ACKNOWLEDGEMENTS 8

PART 1 **HOW EXERCISE REDUCES PAIN** 9

CHAPTER 1	AN INTRODUCTION TO THERAPEUTIC EXERCISE MECHANISMS 11
CHAPTER 2	STRENGTH, PAIN AND THE BRAIN 29
CHAPTER 3	EXERCISE-INDUCED HYPOALGESIA 41
CHAPTER 4	THE PHYSICAL ACTIVITY PARADOX 57
CHAPTER 5	PLACEBO OR NOCEBO: PREPARING TO EXERCISE 65
CHAPTER 6	PAIN EDUCATION, COGNITIVE BEHAVIOURAL THERAPY AND MOTIVATIONAL INTERVIEWING 83
CHAPTER 7	REHABILITATION CONFLICT 109
CHAPTER 8	THE PRINCIPLES OF TRAINING 2.0 117
CHAPTER 9	MOTIVATION AND ADHERENCE 131

PART 2 **REGIONAL REHABILITATION** 141

CHAPTER 10	EXERCISE FOR ANKLE PAIN 143
CHAPTER 11	EXERCISE FOR KNEE PAIN 163
CHAPTER 12	EXERCISE FOR HIP PAIN 187
CHAPTER 13	EXERCISE FOR BACK PAIN 201
CHAPTER 14	EXERCISE FOR SHOULDER PAIN 231
CHAPTER 15	EXERCISE FOR NECK PAIN 249

PREFACE

Exercise is a powerful tool that has been proven to be an effective rehabilitation strategy. However, it is often misunderstood and can lead to disappointment when carefully selected exercises fail to provide relief for persistent musculoskeletal conditions. This book aims to identify what really impacts exercise outcomes and present helpful clinical ideas, tools, and concepts that improve clinical results.

At a time when physical and manual therapists are pursuing bolt-on training courses to allow them to offer rehabilitation services, we are seeing the emergence of two streams of research. The first stream, which could be described as the performance stream, traditionally serves strength trainers and performance coaches and focuses on performance outcomes that include strength, muscular endurance, and other objective measures of performance that would likely improve athletic ability. The second stream, which could be described as the clinical stream, is often concerned with subjective measures of pain and related clinical outcome measures, often less tangible but superior in their importance to the patient in pain.

This book has been written for my past and future students and fellow practitioners. As physiotherapy, sports therapy, chiropractic, and osteopathy students seek to learn how exercise can be used for pain management, this book aims to provide the information you need in a readable, digestible, affordable, and clinically useful way.

Exercise is not just one modality; it is many things wrapped into one intervention. This book aims to explain the different aspects of exercise and provide insights on how to use exercise effectively in clinical practice. I hope that this book will help you achieve successful pain relief from exercise and provide you with the necessary tools to improve clinical outcomes.

Wishing you the very best in the clinic and beyond.

Daniel Lawrence MCSP

ACKNOWLEDGEMENTS

Thank you to my wife Kim Lawrence for everything she does to support my work, including modelling for the book's photographs.

Sonia Cutler, medical copy-editor, who returned to work with me again on my latest book. I look forward to working with Sonia again soon.

Richard Draisey, photographer and videographer for @ThePhysioChannel (YouTube) and Physio Books Ltd.

David Redondo for bringing it all together including the cover design.

PART 1

HOW EXERCISE REDUCES PAIN

Part 1 of the book covers the science behind why exercise can reduce pain and what to do when it does not. It also introduces theories applicable to the whole body as well as localised dysfunctions. I discuss the research relating to the systemic effects of exercise and review the fundamental changes that occur within body systems to help with pain relief.

One of the emergent themes is that specificity of exercise selection is not as important when the goals are pain relief and function compared to a sports setting where goals are performance-based. This is an overlooked factor, especially during the recent uptake of strength and conditioning knowledge and training by therapists looking to offer their clients extended care beyond passive treatment for pain relief.

While there is evidence to support the notion that specificity in exercise selection is not important for pain relief, it would be poor practice to overlook the specific requirements of the individual and their physical abilities and preferences.

CHAPTER 1

AN INTRODUCTION TO THERAPEUTIC EXERCISE MECHANISMS

INTRODUCTION

As this book aims to explain, exercise is not just one modality; rather, it is many things wrapped into one intervention. At its core, it is proven and evidence-based. This should not be confused with guaranteed because even the best exercises do not work for every patient. This book aims to identify these outcome influencers and present helpful clinical ideas, as well as tools and concepts to improve the clinical rehabilitation of the client.

The aim of this chapter is to introduce the many ways in which therapeutic exercise is proposed to work. Therapeutic exercise is prescribed to reduce pain and improve physical function after injuries and to manage persistent pain conditions. It also serves to restore 'movement confidence' and facilitate normal psychological well-being, which is often influenced by social function and the ability to participate actively in everyday life.

Throughout my early career, it was normal for most people to be given their exercises as 3 sets of 10. This physiotherapy exercise mantra has now been updated and improved thanks to many excellent textbooks, online courses and educators, all sharing the important principles of strength and conditioning. To be clear, 3 sets of 10 is not wrong but it is like a 'cheese sandwich'; it is better than nothing but there is substantial room for improvement and variety.

At a time when manual therapists are becoming increasingly aware of the effectiveness and evidence base for exercise rehabilitation, and are pursuing bolt-on training modules to allow them to offer rehabilitation services, we are seeing the emergence of two streams of research.

The first stream has traditionally served strength trainers and performance coaches and focuses on performance outcomes that include strength, muscular endurance and other objective measures of performance, which would likely improve athletic ability. This first stream could be described as the performance stream.

The second stream of research could be described as the clinical stream. This also looks at performance measures but they are always coupled with subjective measures of pain and related clinical outcome measures, which are often less tangible but superior in their importance to the patient.

At the time of writing this book, I witnessed what I believed to be an unbalanced focus on the performance stream and not enough focus on the clinical stream. If you are rehabilitating a patient from an acute injury or tackling a persistent pain problem, then your aims and objectives will differ from those of a performance coach who is typically aiming to improve an athlete's performance. Clinicians can learn a lot from strength and conditioning coaches, but it is important to realise that the principles of training are only one of many ingredients required to achieve successful pain relief using exercise. Clinicians and performance coaches require different outcomes from exercise, while also sharing some other outcomes. Exercise for pain relief is different than exercise for performance. If we only rely on strength and conditioning principles when helping our patients, we will invariably fail to achieve good clinical outcomes.

The relationship between pain and tissue damage has been extensively studied and discussed. We now know that they can be independent variables. A minor injury can be perceived as very painful while a large traumatic lesion can be painless. Pain can also be reported in the absence of tissue damage.

We know less about the relationship between pain and strength. The simple premise is that strengthening muscles and getting stronger is one of the common aims and measurable goals of rehabilitation. The other goal is pain reduction. Therefore, it is often assumed that increased strength will reduce pain. We might assume that increased strength allows more joint support, improved control of ground reaction force and easier function; however, evidence suggests that these factors may be independent of reported pain relief. There is more to strengthening than increased strength measures and peripheral tissue adaptation. Reductions in reported pain can occur without increases in strength. Similarly, improvements in strength can occur without reductions in pain. Thus, they are independent variables and highlight that exercise for pain relief is not just a case of getting stronger.

As an example, think of a patient with knee pain who is also reporting difficulty descending stairs. Knee pain could be due to tissue damage or could be caused by peripheral sensitisation or both of these. The patient may also be thinking negatively about the knee pain, catastrophising about the possible outcome and becoming hypervigilant of any sensations arising from the knee leading to central sensitisation and guarding behaviour. There may also be pain-increasing social influence from social media or from speaking to friends or colleagues about their knee. This social influence is called vicarious learning or social contagion, that is, well-meaning but misunderstood. Professionals can be the cause of such vicarious learning or social contagion. Thus, what the professional explains is often not what the patient interprets, especially when medical terminology is used.

Therefore, we can see that the causes of knee pain, weakness and dysfunction could be due to multiple factors, that is, between individuals and within individuals, during their recovery.

One dysfunction mechanism could be muscle atrophy of the quadricep muscles, but there is more to muscle than size (e.g. cross-sectional area); for example, loss of motor control and excessive, irrational and debilitating fear of pain from movement (kinesiophobia) can cause habitual tissue unloading and weakening. Under these scenarios, pain education can be a powerful way of reducing pain and improving strength and function by making the patient less fearful and more willing to load.

Pain and dysfunction can also scramble the acuity of sensory input from the painful region and reduce motor output. These changes have been noted in the somatosensory cortex of the brain. The cortical representation of a joint or function can become less clear and 'smudging' may occur. Smudging occurs when the size or precision of neuronal firing patterns related to a functional movement are reduced. Smudging does not cause pain but often a mismatch between sensory input and motor output correlate with increased pain; correcting the interpretation of sensory information has been shown to commonly occur alongside pain reduction. We will return to this topic twice more in the book, that is, in Chapter 8 when we look at specificity and when we consider precision training, and in Chapter 13 when we look at low back pain exercise.

Strengthening also offers an element of exposure. The patient is exposed to movements that they were avoiding and therefore learn that they can tolerate those movements, manage any associated pain and not experience a decline in their well-being. Exposure is not necessarily about completing a task without pain; it is about experiencing pain, accepting it and reducing its inherent threat.

Even a basic exercise stimulus could foster improved motor control, for example, stimulating the muscles around a joint to contract faster, which aids dissipation of rapid loading forces. A reduction in pain coupled with pain education can also help to put any magnetic resonance imaging (MRI), X-ray or other imaging results into context, allowing the patient to be less worried about some of the structural reports that have been communicated to them. The power of negative verbal information should not be ignored. If comprehended, words can convert non-nociceptive stimulation into pain to the same level as a painful stimulus (Colloca et al., 2008). Thus, words matter!

Another interesting topic we discuss in more depth in Chapter 3 is exercise-induced hypoalgesia (EIH). EIH can occur with both cardiovascular exercise and strengthening. EIH causes a short period of reduced-pain sensitivity (hypoalgesia) after exercising. EIH also occurs via multiple central pathways and can therefore be very broad in its effects; thus, you do not need to exercise the joint that hurts to experience hypoalgesia. Whole-body exercise could be performed for isolated joint pathologies or, more specifically, the opposite joint could be exercised to reduce the perceived pain in the injured joint. This offers some helpful tools in the clinic. We will now take a closer look at some of these proposed mechanisms.

PHYSICAL CHANGES

In making the case for exercise for pain relief, we can appreciate that therapeutic exercise is about so much more than simply improving strength output, hypertrophy and physical adaptations. It is, however, important to maintain awareness of these physiological adaptations and appreciate their role in a rehabilitation setting. Research often measures maximum voluntary isometric contraction (MVIC), which is the maximum voluntary contraction the patient can produce isometrically against a resistance measuring tool. It is important to note the 'voluntary' element of the test because the contractile capacity of a muscle is modulated by the brain and motor output. If the muscle was directly stimulated, a higher-strength contraction may occur and this is often delivered by superimposing an electrical current to the contractile tissue. Can you see how the voluntary element could easily be influenced by injury concerns, pain and general willingness to perform the MVIC test?

Another measure of muscle function is the rate of force development (RFD), which is a measure of contraction speed. For example, if the RFD is reduced in the quadriceps, then the muscles' ability to absorb ground reaction forces and allow an efficient gait pattern is reduced, and the patient may report that their knee feels like it is giving way. There is a reduced RFD in the gastrocnemius–soleus complex of individuals with Achilles tendinopathy (Azevedo et al., 2009), which reduces the efficiency of the tendon spring mechanism but may also serve a protective purpose as tendon stress is reduced in favour of a prolonged muscular effort.

As well as normalising RFD to dissipate ground reaction forces and protect joints, a feedforward mechanism stabilises the central part of the body ahead of peripheral limb movement. For example, in the upper body, the muscles around the neck contract ahead of shoulder movement to stabilise the cervical spine (Falla et al., 2004). This has also been reported in the lumbar spine (Leinonen et al., 2001). Any dysfunction of this feedforward preparatory movement pattern typically normalises quickly after injury but can continue in chronic pain states (Falla et al., 2004), with motor control training showing the potential to restore dysfunctions (Tsao & Hodges, 2007).

Thus, restoration of function requires more than just pure strength; it requires normalisation of contraction speed and coordination with other synergist muscle groups.

BUILDING RESERVE CAPACITY

We need a maximal and endurance strength capacity in excess of our normal daily demands. If we are only as strong as our normal daily tasks require, then we have no reserve capacity, no buffer zone and no extra strength to protect from overload and injury. For example, if walking up the stairs independently and pain-free after a knee operation requires 90% of a patient's maximum strength, then, by definition, they are working very hard and they do not have much reserve or buffer left in the system. They would reach a level of fatigue sooner, experience reduced muscle coordination sooner and be more susceptible to overload with only a 10% strength reserve. This concept not only helps us understand the efficacy of improving strength output; it also serves as a way of explaining the importance of strength rehabilitation to our clients. If we can achieve a modest increase in maximal strength, then we can easily double an individual's strength reserve during daily tasks, offering injury protection in the form of increased capacity and resilience. In Chapter 13, we look at resilience in relation to lumbar spine rehabilitation because it involves more than just maximal strength capacity.

IMPROVED MOVEMENT, POSTURE AND BALANCE

Exercise interventions may also provide an opportunity to explore new ways of movement that are more comfortable due to redistribution of load between different joints or improved movement ranges from desensitised stretch reflexes that allow day-to-day flexibility functions, such as putting shoes and socks on, to become much easier. Movement may also be less threatening due to altered perception of salient sensations through increased knowledge and education.

Reduced resting muscle tone, which occurs after exercise, allows for reduced bracing and hyperstability, often reported by the patient as tension felt around the cervical and lumbar spine.

This could be described to the patient using the clenched fist visual metaphor. If you are experiencing wrist pain, making a fist and tensing the wrist may increase wrist pain and stiffness; when you then try to move while maintaining a clenched fist, the wrist will probably click and grind. The client could then be told that muscle tension can be a common reason for the clicking, grinding and pain felt in the neck. With cervical muscles in a state of increased tone, they may worsen the dysfunction. Explaining this to clients allows them to appreciate that relaxing the muscles around the painful region is often a prerequisite to increase range of motion. In the clinic, I occasionally find that clients brace themselves into what they consider good postures, whereas doing this may actually delay their recovery.

Posture may be a target for rehabilitation. While there is a lack of evidence linking posture to pain, posture is still a variable that matters and both clients and many clinicians still hold strong posture beliefs. Posture can influence many parts of our body, for example, our posture can change our breathing mechanics. Maintaining different postures can also load the tissues and cause discomfort, suggesting that the onset of pain is due to a lack of movement rather than a specific posture. Recent evidence suggests that postural changes can improve regional function (Ludwig et al., 2018; Suzuki et al., 2019).

I believe it is sensible to advise clients positively and pragmatically on posture as part of an exercise for pain relief plan. Dispelling common misconceptions, such as sitting up straight or pulling the shoulders back and down, is important; instead, one should instil the notion that relaxed postures are not harmful and a more relaxed prolonged positioning is probably a better pain-reducing strategy than sitting up straight for hours on end. Of course, it is better to be up and moving regularly; however, many sedentary individuals do not achieve this in reality.

Various exercise approaches can restore balance and balance problems are not limited to older individuals. The research indicates that common ankle inversion injuries can cause a decline in single-leg stance balance in both injured and non-injured legs (Donovan & Hertel, 2012). The three systems that contribute to balance are visual, vestibular and proprioceptive; any exercise that targets at least one of these systems has the potential to improve balance. Functional balance training typically stimulates all of these systems and we look at some specific methods in the chapter about ankle rehabilitation (Chapter 10).

PSYCHOLOGICAL MECHANISMS

Exercise can influence psychological variables such as kinesiophobia, catastrophising and pain perception; historically these have been seen as vague, less defined secondary benefits. It is now increasingly likely that these are the primary determinants of the success of exercise for pain relief. Success may be less determined by exercise repetitions or the biomechanics of physical training. Instead, getting patients to understand their thoughts applied to the exercise endeavour, getting them to understand what and why they are performing certain physical manoeuvres and having positive realistic outcome expectations may have a larger impact on the final outcome.

Whenever possible, we want to create situations where patients have a positive experience of exercise. One that enhances their mood, changes their perception and creates a positive outcome expectation. This can influence pain and it is a form of latent inhibition. Latent inhibition is not limited to exercise outcome; it is a term from classical psychological conditioning that refers to when pre-exposure to a stimulus without consequence impedes subsequent responses because a consequence is not expected based on the previous experience. In a rehabilitation context, if an individual has had a previous positive experience of exercise, then they are more likely to expect and therefore achieve positive recovery the second or third or fourth time round, for example. This is latent inhibition in action; previous positive outcomes (or lack of a negative outcome) help to reduce pain with current experiences. The opposite scenario, where patients have had a negative experience of exercise rehabilitation, can cause a negative expectation. Many of my new clients show reluctance to try exercises based on their previous exercise failure. There is a way forward with these patients using the strategies outlined in this book.

Most of an exercise for pain relief plan will be completed by the patient independently and this creates an opportunity to gain a sense of control, improving confidence and self-efficacy. As we discuss in the chapter about motivation and adherence (Chapter 9), we may need to nurture this internal locus of control through more patient contact and guidance initially to help manage pain flare-ups and typical symptom fluctuations. Support at these key times will avoid learned helplessness through education and guidance provided at a time when it is needed most.

Some patients require more intensive support than others, particularly those at risk of chronicity. In Chapter 13, we discuss the recommended level of support for subgroups of individuals with back pain.

EXPOSURE THERAPY

Exposure therapy can be one of the key mechanisms underpinning the success of exercise for pain relief. Guided rehabilitation gives the patient exposure to movements that they may have been avoiding. Exposure provides an opportunity to extinguish previous maladaptive beliefs that certain movements and loading could be painful by providing a form of experiential reassurance.

Exposure therapy is often misunderstood in individuals with chronic pain. Pain during the task is acceptable and exposure therapy is not always aimed at reducing pain; instead, it can be used to reduce the threat value of pain and improve pain tolerance as individuals learn that pain does not equal damage and that they can tolerate activity-related pain without lasting consequences or a deterioration in their condition. This behavioural switch from avoidance to engagement can often lead to more positive changes as the individual returns to normal activities while being able to manage and tolerate pain rather than resting and avoiding tasks until the pain is fully resolved, which unfortunately does not occur in individuals with chronic, persistent pain.

I once assessed a client who experienced back pain lifting something at work and had been sitting watching TV for 6 months waiting for their back to recover before going back to work. They were not an easy client to work with and I wish I had this book back then to help me manage them more effectively; however, they were probably one of the catalysts for researching the content for this book.

Exercise exposure also helps to create robust coping strategies so the individual can find ways to self-manage their condition, learn how much activity and load they can tolerate and how they can modulate their perception of pain using management strategies that may include psychological methods such as visualisation, distraction and relaxation techniques.

REMOVAL OF 'EX-CONSEQUENTIA' REASONING

Ex-consequentia reasoning has been reported in behavioural science anxiety research. It refers to situations where a person feels the sensation of anxiety and determines that there must be something real to be anxious about. This may be relatable in the clinic when an individual feels an atypical sensation from a joint like clunking, clicking, grinding or pain and concludes that this must be due to structural joint damage. In this book, we discuss this again and introduce methods to quash these barriers to rehabilitation.

EXERCISE EFFECTS ON THE CENTRAL NERVOUS SYSTEM

Exercise has multiple effects on the central nervous system (CNS); although much less researched than peripheral adaptations, recent testing methods like functional MRI have facilitated a better understanding of the CNS response to exercise. Athletic research primarily focuses on central fatigue mechanisms, while clinical research is concerned with the regulation of circadian rhythms, central metabolic functions and stress responses. Dysregulation of these functions is common in psychiatric conditions like depression and common neurological conditions such as Alzheimer's disease.

Regular exercise has a protective effect on the brain, protecting or delaying cognitive decline. In a clinical setting, a more acute elevation of mood and self-perception supports the success of rehabilitation and a return to normal function. This positive attentional focus and stimulus from exercise also promotes neural plasticity and is supportive of cortical reorganisation.

One interesting variable that may influence the CNS response to exercise is whether it is forced or voluntary. This has been concluded primarily from murine studies, with mice and rats completing either voluntary or forced wheel running (Cook et al., 2013). Forced exercise is thought to have an additional stress component. In Chapter 3, we look at forced versus voluntary exercise with reference to both murine and human studies. This may be another differentiator between performance training and exercise for pain relief because performance training involves a forced effort; in a clinical setting, a self-paced exercise may be preferred and forced intensity may cause a negative response to exercise. In the author's opinion, there is not enough evidence to apply this principle rigidly to rehabilitation for pain reduction; perhaps, it may depend on personality type and the individual's exercise preferences, which are discussed in Chapter 7.

One factor that can affect overall well-being and recovery is sleep quality, typically regulated by a well-functioning circadian clock. There are many reasons why this rhythm can be disrupted after pain and injury, including loss of training routine, occupational routine and chronic stress. Positively scheduled exercise can contribute to improved sleep rhythms (Hughes & Piggins, 2012). Improving sleep quality can be hugely influential for patients with persistent pain. In the clinic, I have seen a link between sleep disturbance and people's ability to manage pain.

EXERCISE EFFECTS ON CNS OUTPUT

Reduced strength can be centrally mediated by cortical inhibition; if the brain is not fully engaging the motor system, then the contractile capacity of the skeletal muscle tissue will not be fully used. This would have a protective function to reduce tissue stress where structural damage has occurred; however, this motor dampening can perpetuate beyond structural repair and lead to strength deficits. In the clinic, this would present as apprehension when loading, for example, a limp or more subtle deficits, such as reduced lower-limb control when descending stairs.

From a rehabilitation perspective, the role of the CNS in modulating strength has historically been overlooked. Restoration of cortical representation, so that areas of the body have normal cortical mapping in the brain, influences not only the skill components of our movement but also the total strength output. Thus, a more precise neuronal pattern representing a movement will improve both the MVIC and the precision of the movement. We look at some specific research in Chapter 2 where we delve deeper into the link between strength, pain and the brain.

DESCENDING INHIBITION

There are three main systems that may cause or collectively contribute to descending inhibition:

1. the endogenous opioid system;
2. the endocannabinoid system; and
3. the serotonergic system.

These systems provide proposed mechanisms for EIH, something that we discuss in more depth in Chapter 3, as well as exercise-induced hyperalgesia, which is an unfavourable increase in pain after exercise and is common in certain subgroups of individuals.

IMMUNE SYSTEM CHANGES

Depending on the level and intensity of the exercise, we can also induce immune system changes with the release of anti-inflammatory cytokines that can offset an inflammatory response. The intensity of the exercise is influential on the stress response, with the release of adrenaline and cortisol having a positive effect on pain mechanisms. As already mentioned, the difference between voluntary and forced exercise can influence the inflammatory effects, with forced exercise and associated stress increasing inflammation in mice (Cook et al., 2013).

A common theory suggests that a vigorous bout of exercise can temporarily suppress immune function. Campbell and Turner (2018) reported that limited evidence supports this theory and exercise probably has a positive effect on the immune system in both the short and long term. The research reviewed in Chapter 4 also provides an interesting theory that low levels of continued occupational physical activity may lead to continued asymptomatic increases in inflammatory cytokines due to continued and externally paced activity (Holtermann et al., 2017).

CONCLUSION

This opening chapter should have increased your awareness of the multiple potential mechanisms that account for the pain relief experienced from rehabilitation exercise. Rather than viewing this as an academic exercise to understand the complexity of exercise for pain relief mechanisms, this book aims to help you harness this understanding so that you can then assess and manipulate the variables in the clinical setting to improve the outcomes for your clients.

REFERENCES

Azevedo LB, Lambert MI, Vaughan CL, O'Connor CM, Schwellnus MP (2009). Biomechanical variables associated with Achilles tendinopathy in runners. *Br J Sports Med* 43:288–292.

Campbell JP, Turner JE (2018). Debunking the myth of exercise-induced immune suppression: redefining the impact of exercise on immunological health across the lifespan. *Front Immunol* 9:648.

Colloca L, Sigaudo M, Benedetti F (2008). The role of learning in nocebo and placebo effects. *Pain* 136:211–218.

Cook MD, Martin SA, Williams C, et al. (2013). Forced treadmill exercise training exacerbates inflammation and causes mortality while voluntary wheel training is protective in a mouse model of colitis. *Brain Behav Immun* 33:46–56.

Donovan L, Hertel J (2012). A new paradigm for rehabilitation of patients with chronic ankle instability. *Phys Sportsmed* 40:41–51.

Falla D, Jull G, Hodges PW (2004). Feedforward activity of the cervical flexor muscles during voluntary arm movements is delayed in chronic neck pain. *Exp Brain Res* 157:43–48.

Holtermann A, Krause N, van der Beek AJ, Straker L (2017). The physical activity paradox: six reasons why occupational physical activity (OPA) does not confer the cardiovascular health benefits that leisure time physical activity does. *Br J Sports Med* 52:149–150.

Hughes AT, Piggins HD (2012). Feedback actions of locomotor activity to the circadian clock. *Prog Brain Res* 199:305–336.

Leinonen V, Kankaanpää M, Luukkonen M, et al. (2001). Disc herniation-related back pain impairs feed-forward control of paraspinal muscles. *Spine* 26:E367–E372.

Ludwig O, Kelm J, Hammes A, Schmitt E, Fröhlich M (2018). Targeted athletic training improves the neuromuscular performance in terms of body posture from adolescence to adulthood–long-term study over 6 years. *Front Physiol* 9:1620.

Suzuki Y, Muraki T, Sekiguchi Y, et al. (2019). Influence of thoracic posture on scapulothoracic and glenohumeral motions during eccentric shoulder external rotation. *Gait Posture* 67:207–212.

Tsao H, Hodges PW (2007). Immediate changes in feedforward postural adjustments following voluntary motor training. *Exp Brain Res* 18:537–546.

CHAPTER 2

STRENGTH, PAIN AND THE BRAIN

INTRODUCTION

This chapter makes the case that exercise rehabilitation is not all about strength; therefore, a poor correlation between pain reduction and strength increase is suggested. However, measuring strength is useful and motivating, so we certainly should not invalidate measures of improved strength. Improved strength in the absence of pain relief is still a positive outcome and one that may promote exercise adherence, which inherently provides some future relief from pain.

This chapter identifies the more central adaptations in the brain that influence and are influenced by strength training and how such adaptations can alter motor and strength output. We also look into matters most relevant for pain relief and discuss relevant research. Where research is lacking, we identify clues within the research that can guide our future rehabilitation plans.

Musculoskeletal injury usually causes reported and detectable muscle weakness, commonly termed muscle inhibition. Such deficits are typically measured as reduced maximal voluntary isometric contraction (MVIC) and reduced rate of force development (RFD), which is a measure of contraction speed. We might assume that this is due to local muscle weakness at a peripheral level. In this chapter, I argue that after-injury muscle inhibition is most probably a centrally mediated phenomenon.

In the early stages after an injury, centrally mediated strength loss serves a protective purpose. Reduced contraction power protects recovering tissues from excessive loading, for example, falling to the ground when you roll your ankle serves to immediately offload your ankle and prevents further damage to the tissues. Another example might be reduced load tolerance through your knee after a fall, which causes an antalgic but protective offloading limp. These adaptive responses are helpful and serve our recovery. At some point, and the exact point is hard to define, being more of a phase than a certain moment in time, muscle inhibition becomes maladaptive and can continue in the absence of pain.

In a clinical setting, we often identify muscle weakness (reduced MVIC) from the area reported as painful. This would typically be detected using a simple manual push test where the client pushes a limb against your hand; by comparing both sides, you may determine a strength deficit. Perhaps you have more scientific measuring tools but that is not significant for the theory I am explaining here. If we assume that muscle weakness is purely a peripheral issue and disregard the brain's influence while continuing with peripherally targeted rehabilitation, then we would be taking a very limited rehabilitation path.

Understanding how individuals respond to strengthening exercises is different than understanding how athletes respond to strengthening. While many of the processes are the same, some of the variables considered negligible by strength coaches may in fact be primary mechanisms for functional recovery and analgesia in clinical practice.

It is commonly agreed that exercise-based rehabilitation has one of the highest efficacies for reducing musculoskeletal pain from a variety of causes. However, our knowledge of the mechanisms is still unclear. Many factors can contribute to reduced muscle performance, from the physical size of the muscle, usually referred to as cross-sectional area, physiological fatigue from continued hypertonus, changes in muscle fibre type and delayed contraction speed; perhaps less discussed and understood are the psychological and social influences that receive much needed attention in this chapter.

SETTING THE SCENE WITH THE RESEARCH

A significant systematic review by Steiger et al. (2012) asked the following question in the title: Is a positive clinical outcome after exercise therapy for chronic non-specific low back pain contingent upon a corresponding improvement in the targeted aspect(s) of performance?

This was an in-depth review that can really challenge some people's long-held beliefs and assumptions. It may present some challenging conclusions for some readers but that is what makes a good read!

Let us familiarise ourselves with some of the data they used in their systematic review. Sixteen studies with a total of 1476 participants were included. The 16 studies included a wide range of interventions, outcome measures and group selection procedures. The durations of follow-up were also very varied. This wide variance in the 16 studies led to a broad range of results that reduced the ability to form firm conclusions.

Next, let us review some of their results. There was minimal evidence supporting the association between pain and changes in objective performance measures. Steiger et al. (2012) collated the results to look for the following potential correlations between pain and functional disability and the relationship with the following performance measures: sagittal; rotational; lateral mobility; trunk extension and trunk flexion strength; and back muscle endurance.

Many of the studies reviewed did not report a pain–performance relationship in the data. In statistics, this relationship is called the correlation coefficient. A correlation coefficient of 0 means that no relationship has been identified between two variables like pain and range of flexion, for example. A perfect relationship would be either +1 or −1. After combining the results from the different studies, the correlations were all low to very low. For example, 3 studies correlated pain and sagittal (flexion and extension) mobility with an overall correlation of −0.009 (very low). Four studies looked at the relationship between pain and spinal extension strength, with an overall correlation of 0.262 (low).

The authors concluded that there is no convincing evidence that changes in objective measures like range of motion or strength are strongly associated with reductions in pain or disability. When reduced pain and improved strength occur together, it could be argued that reduced pain and improved strength occur coincidentally. Another theory is that other contributing components of recovery are stimulated by exercise therapy. These could be the psychological, social and more centrally mediated neurological components that we discuss and expand on in this book, including the importance of the therapist–client relationship, which is deemed an important determinant of outcome (Hall et al., 2010).

Next, we review a well-written and interesting single-case report of an individual who received cognitive functional therapy for chronic non-specific neck pain (Meziat-Filho et al., 2018). This is a very interesting study because the individual presented with limited cervical extension and rotation during the initial assessment. The next contact with this individual was at the 1-month follow-up, when they reported restoration of the previously painful cervical extension and rotation and overall improvement to an almost asymptomatic status. So far, this case history reads as unremarkable. The interesting part is that the individual did not practice the extension and rotation exercises at home. The report states that they only performed them under guidance at the initial appointment. So not only was their home exercise regime not specific to their dysfunctions, it was also void of the actual target movements. In reality, we can assume they would have extended and rotated their neck during normal daily activities to at least a low level but there was no focused or repetitive performance of these two actions.

The authors suggested that the recovery was probably mediated by a change from an initial negative belief to a more positive one, plus some mitigation of pain hypervigilance (Meziat-Filho et al., 2018). The positive experience from even just one guided exercise session would have allowed an exposure learning experience and an appreciation that the previously avoided cervical motions of extension and rotation could be performed without negative consequences, thus reducing kinesiophobia through a latent inhibition effect. In truth, the mechanisms that underlie a successful outcome could be many other things and explained in different ways; however, regardless of how this case study is interpreted, it further strengthens the notion of non-specificity and the multi-system mechanisms of exercise for pain relief.

As we continue the topic of strength, pain and the brain, we can begin to appreciate the power of the brain in regulating strength output, just as we know that it regulates pain perception. Both strength and pain could be described as brain outputs. Although you can produce strength through direct electrical muscle stimulation, without the need for brain output, this is rather useless from a useable functional perspective.

The next study by Clark and colleagues (2014), included three groups of uninjured and healthy people. Two groups had their non-dominant wrist and hand voluntarily immobilised in a rigid cast for 4 weeks. The other group served as the control group and were not immobilised. Of the two immobilised groups, one group completed 52 imaginary maximal muscle contractions 5 times per week. These were not isometric and only 'imagined' contractions. To make sure they were not actually contracting, electromyography readings were monitored to detect any surges in electrical activity in the muscles. The other group remained immobilised and did not complete these sessions. After 4 weeks, strength loss in the imagined contraction group was 50% lower than the group that did not imagine any wrist flexor contractions.

This suggests that there is a very important cortical element to strengthening and it is not simply about hypertrophy, peripheral adaptations and the transmission of contractile messages through the motor pathways.

The role of the primary motor cortex and other higher-order cortical regions are seldom acknowledged as being a significant factor in determining muscle strength. The primary motor cortex has historically been seen as more involved with movement coordination and skill acquisition than maximum force generation (Adkins et al., 2006; Remple et al., 2001).

This is why simple cognitions like mental imagery, which have been shown to activate the primary motor cortex, can be highly effective at increasing muscle strength through improved voluntary activation.

Pearson and colleagues (2009) measured the maximal voluntary isometric neck forces in a group of individuals with whiplash-associated disorder and in a group of healthy individuals. They also assessed for links between strength measurements and pain, kinesiophobia and catastrophising in the group with the whiplash-associated disorder.

The results unsurprisingly showed that the group with the whiplash-associated disorder had reduced strength outputs, specifically extension, retraction and left lateral rotation. The results also showed no significant association between neck strength and measures of disability, kinesiophobia and catastrophising. On the surface, this does not support the theory of strength being mediated by psychosocial factors. However, if we look at the results of this study in more detail, an interesting phenomenon occurs. Between sessions 1 and 2, many individuals demonstrated measurable increases in their neck strength outputs; the changes were large enough to be true measures and not measurement errors. So why were they able to produce more force? The authors suggested that the experience of the first testing session made them realise that it was not going to cause their condition to worsen and thus led them to willingly produce more effort at the second testing session.

DISCUSSION

Historically, it was assumed that improvements in strength were the cause of reduced pain; however, the research presented in this chapter fails to identify this causative link. Reduced pain is suggested to be mediated more centrally (Steiger et al., 2012). This might also explain why the clinical exercise literature does not support specific exercises or training parameters and positive outcomes have been reported from a wide range of physical activity interventions. On balance, specific exercise interventions also yield very varied results for pathology-matched groups.

For example, no particular type of exercise therapy for low back pain is presently considered to be superior to another. As we discuss throughout this book, this may be because the exercise is not actually producing benefits by just improving strength measures. In fact, if pain reduction and strength can be improved by reducing the threat of movement, this might explain why even stretching exercises can improve strength (Khalil et al., 1992). This suggests that any kind of movement therapy, not just stretching, could create improved strength outcomes. It would be incorrect to assume that stretching improves strength as a general concept. Instead, suggesting that any input that corrects the central drivers of motor output could induce strength increases is a more plausible inference. These inputs could be physical, cognitive or possibly augmented by a mix of both.

Exercise for pain relief requires more than just instructing strengthening exercises. The individual's recovering joint and surrounding supportive musculature may already have a good structural capacity for load tolerance and may only require a moderate exercise stimulus to restore central drive and engage the motor neuron pools to activate the peripheral contractile tissue. Perhaps, most importantly, the individual needs help to overcome any psychological barriers to loading the tissues, which may include barriers such as fear of causing harm, social barriers such as a well-meaning spouse who advocates too much rest, and physical barriers such as difficulty selecting an appropriate exercise or activity. If the changes we are looking for are more centrally mediated, then we can focus less on exercise parameters like repetitions and sets and more on the individual's thoughts and cognitions of why an exercise is being performed and how it can help them. This is a matter of rebalancing the exercise focus and not disregarding the importance of the exercise principles we cover in Chapter 8.

TOOLS FOR THE CLINIC

The clinical utility of this information could be as follows:

- Strength can be targeted centrally with reframing tactics like pain education, cognitive behavioural therapy and mental imagery.
- Mental imagery can be used in isolation or to augment early movement interventions. For example, the individual could move through a small range of motion but imagine they are moving through a large range of motion. They could also imagine increased load demands before they are applied in reality.
- Pain education could include attempts to destructuralise the individual's beliefs of the cause of their problem, for example, by teaching that not all pain needs a structural cause and that imaging findings may just be normal variations or normal age-related changes.
- Exercise exposure can provide an educational opportunity to reduce kinesiophobia through experiential learning.

CONCLUSION

After the introduction of these studies and the theories discussed therein, we can appreciate that strength is controlled by the brain; therefore, like pain, we can target the brain to improve, restore or remove barriers to regain strength after injury. This knowledge also opens up new avenues for the use of strength training in persistent conditions based on the understanding that the aims and outcomes are much broader than peripheral adaptations and increases in strength measures. The very process of training offers rehabilitation opportunities beyond physical performance.

If we downgrade the significance of physical performance deficits like strength and flexibility and instead focus on creating a positive exercise experience with opportunities for cognitive restructuring, then we may achieve greater and more frequent success with our exercise interventions.

REFERENCES

Adkins DL, Boychuk J, Remple MS, Kleim JA (2006). Motor training induces experience-specific patterns of plasticity across motor cortex and spinal cord. *J Appl Physiol* 101:1776–1782.

Clark BC, Mahato NK, Nakazawa M, Law TD, Thomas JS (2014). The power of the mind: the cortex as a critical determinant of muscle strength/weakness. *J Neurophysiol* 112:3219–3226.

Hall AM, Ferreira PH, Maher CG, Latimer J, Ferreira ML (2010). The influence of the therapist–patient relationship on treatment outcome in physical rehabilitation: a systematic review. *Phys Ther* 90:1099–1110.

Khalil TM, Asfour SS, Martinez LM, Waly SM, Rosomoff RS, Rosomoff HL (1992). Stretching in the rehabilitation of low-back pain patients. *Spine* 17:311–317.

Meziat-Filho N, Lima M, Fernandez J, Reis FJJ (2018). Cognitive Functional Therapy (CFT) for chronic non-specific neck pain. *J Bodyw Mov Ther* 22:32–36.

Pearson, I., Reichert, A., De Serres, S. J., Dumas, J.-P., & Côté, J. N. (2009). Maximal Voluntary Isometric Neck Strength Deficits in Adults With Whiplash-Associated Disorders and Association With Pain and Fear of Movement. Journal of Orthopaedic & Sports Physical Therapy, 39(3), 179–187.

Remple MS, Bruneau RM, VandenBerg PM, Goertzen C, Kleim JA (2001). Sensitivity of cortical movement representations to motor experience: evidence that skill learning but not strength training induces cortical reorganization. *Behav Brain Res* 123:133–141.

Steiger F, Wirth B, de Bruin ED, Mannion AF (2012). Is a positive clinical outcome after exercise therapy for chronic non-specific low back pain contingent upon a corresponding improvement in the targeted aspect(s) of performance? A systematic review. *Eur Spine J* 21:575–598.

CHAPTER 3

EXERCISE-INDUCED HYPOALGESIA

INTRODUCTION

Around the time of researching for this chapter, I was reading a book called *The Salt Path* by Raynor Winn. This is a true story about the author and her husband, a man called Moth who is diagnosed with corticobasal degeneration, a rare progressive neurological disorder. Moth is prescribed a pain medication called pregabalin, originally developed as an antiseizure epileptic drug. Moth is also advised to 'take it easy'!

Against the medical advice and after a few hundred miles of walking the South West Coast Path in the UK (near my home), carrying everything he owns and accompanied by his wife, he stops taking pregabalin and is experiencing significantly less pain. His wife, the author, notes that the prolonged rhythmic exercise provided by walking all day stimulates the body's natural pain relief mechanisms. Thorén et al. (1990) proposed that this type of rhythmic exercise increases the discharge from mechanosensitive afferent nerve fibres arising from contracting skeletal muscle and activates central opioid systems. What Moth experienced during his walk was exercise-induced hypoalgesia (EIH), a phenomenon with powerful clinical utility and the focus of this chapter.

EXERCISE-INDUCED HYPOALGESIA

EIH can be described as an exercise-induced reduction in pain sensitivity and is a well-documented feature of exercise. This chapter presents the underlying mechanisms in an attempt to understand why some people experience pain relief during and after exercise and why some subgroups of individuals actually experience the opposite effect with increased pain and sensitivity. With these two potential outcomes in mind, we discuss clinical strategies to improve our exercise outcomes for both of these EIH responder and non-responder groups.

EIH is triggered by an increase in blood pressure that stimulates several systems, including the endogenous opioid system (Hoffmann & Thorén, 1988). As discussed later in this chapter, many other systems probably contribute to successful EIH. In terms of neuroanatomy, the periaqueductal grey is considered the control centre for descending inhibition. Descending inhibitory mechanisms are a key component of EIH. The periaqueductal grey is located in the midbrain at the top of the brainstem.

In healthy people, a single bout of aerobic or resistance training leads to a period of successful EIH. However, in some people a single bout of aerobic or resistance training leads to increased sensitivity to pain; this is called exercise-induced hyperalgesia, which is typically termed dysfunctional EIH. This increased pain response (hyperalgesia) is more prevalent in specific populations. We identify these groups and discuss their management in this chapter.

The two clinical questions we need to concern ourselves with are:

1. What is the best way to achieve EIH?
2. How can we manage individuals who present with dysfunctional EIH?

EIH is achieved most effectively with either aerobic exercise at around 70% VO_2 maximum (maximum oxygen consumption) (Koltyn, 2002) or with resistance training (dynamic or isometric) where research indicates that effort levels as low as 10–30% of maximum volitional contraction will suffice if they are sustained to muscular fatigue (Hoeger Bement et al., 2008).

There are identified differences in EIH outcome depending on whether a cardiovascular or resistance stimulus is used. The cardiovascular approach offers a systemic (full-body) analgesia that lasts for about 30 minutes or longer, whereas resistance training facilitates a more localised and shorter-lasting analgesic response (Kosek, Ekholm & Hansson, 1996; Naugle, Fillingim & Riley, 2012). Despite the differences in outcome, both approaches can offer the benefit of EIH. This suggests that we can let our clients choose their preferred mode of exercise.

A knowledge of EIH brings into question the efficacy of the common habit of taking analgesics or anti-inflammatories first thing in the morning or before exercising; individuals may be incorrectly attributing pain relief to the recently ingested medication rather than the EIH resulting from completion of their exercises or even just their less structured physical morning tasks. This type of ritualistic safety behaviour is positively reinforced each time the individual repeats it. Breaking this cycle is a form of exposure therapy, which if successful can provide a powerful learning experience that may reduce analgesia use.

As already mentioned, some individuals experience dysfunctional EIH or exercise-induced hyperalgesia (increased sensitivity to pain). In the clinic, this commonly presents as a symptomatic flare-up after an attempted exercise intervention. You can appreciate the negative impact this would have on motivation and adherence as an initial negative experience of exercise maintains kinesiophobia and exercise avoidance behaviours.

The research indicates that the diagnostic subgroups with the following disorders commonly suffer from dysfunctional EIH:

- fibromyalgia;
- chronic fatigue syndrome, also known as myalgic encephalomyelitis (ME);
- shoulder myalgia;
- painful knee osteoarthritis;
- diabetic neuropathy;
- chronic neck pain; and
- whiplash-associated disorder.

This list covers a wide range of conditions. I would also suggest that any individual with pain sensitivity from suspected diminished central nociceptive processing (central sensitivity) would also have an increased risk of experiencing dysfunctional EIH. This presents a challenging dilemma in the clinic. Do we explain the likelihood of a pain flare-up to these patients and therefore manage expectations, or should we reserve this information until we have tested their response to exercise, and by doing this, avoid setting up a negative expectation that may in part be self-fulfilling? We discuss this further in this chapter.

Interestingly, research indicates that while these subgroups have an increased likelihood of an acute negative response to exercise, other groups show generally positive EIH responses. These include individuals with chronic lower back pain and rheumatoid arthritis. It is interesting to note the difference in response identified in the literature between individuals with neck pain and individuals with lower back pain; both of these conditions have strong biopsychosocial influences and are somewhat similar in this respect.

In the clinic, I have not experienced such a contrast of EIH outcomes between clients with neck pain and clients with low back pain. In the clinic, it is also common for individuals to present with a primary condition that is not associated with dysfunctional EIH but to then report other underlying health issues that may be associated with dysfunctional EIH. While obvious in theory, it may not always be apparent in the clinical setting, especially if underlying issues like fibromyalgia have not yet been identified.

HOW DOES EIH OCCUR?

The mechanisms are theoretical but they include the activation of the following systems:

- endogenous opioid;
- endocannabinoid;
- serotonergic;
- noradrenergic;
- immune; and
- autonomic nervous.

The endogenous opioid system is the most cited descending inhibitory mechanism. However, most studies of this system are done on animals and healthy, pain-free people so there are limitations in the research.

The endocannabinoid system is the most probable non-opioid system to be involved and the presence of cannabinoid receptors in the nociceptive processing areas of the brain and spinal cord suggests that endocannabinoids contribute to the control of pain. Exercise also increases circulating endocannabinoids.

The serotonergic system contributes to the modulation of mood, emotion, sleep and pain. Compared to the other systems, it has received less attention in relation to analgesia but may have a role in the analgesic processes and medications that inhibit the reuptake of serotonin (selective serotonin reuptake inhibitors) could be used to combat dysfunctional EIH.

The noradrenergic system activates during exercise to regulate important functions such as heart rate and glucose metabolism. It may also modulate pain.

The response of the immune system can vary. A positive immune response would cause the release of anti-inflammatory mediators in response to an acute bout of exercise-induced stress. However, this response can sometimes be proinflammatory in patients with persistent pain. Research indicates this may be influenced by whether the exercise is forced or voluntary (Cook, Martin & Williams, 2013).

The autonomic nervous system, also known as the involuntary nervous system, contributes to a wide range of bodily functions to maintain homeostasis. It is also an identified contributor to EIH through the regulation of stress hormones such as noradrenaline and cortisol, which can have an analgesic effect via descending nociceptive inhibition, including at the level of the spinal cord (Millan, 2002).

Other proposed contributing mechanisms include conditioned pain modulation and psychological influences, which are discussed further.

SEX BIAS

The literature suggest that females may be more prone to hyperalgesia than men; in the clinic, it certainly appears that more females present with persistent pain than males. However, a systematic literature review of 10 years of research on sex and experimental pain perception reported that men and women are equal in this respect (Racine et al., 2012). Furthermore, suggesting a sex-specific response to

EIH does not provide a pragmatic management approach and risks excluding many other potential variables.

WHY MIGHT EIH FAIL TO OCCUR?

Possible reasons why EIH may fail to occur have been identified and suggested in the research. They include:

- a family history of chronic pain;
- family environment;
- catastrophising;
- mood disturbance;
- age;
- past experiences;
- level of education;
- social influences;
- exercise perception;
- kinesiophobia;
- forced exercise (versus voluntary); and
- externally paced exercise (versus self-paced).

So, as you can see, there are many factors that could trigger dysfunctional EIH; this offers many opportunities for intervention.

A family history of chronic pain can increase an individual's chances of experiencing persistent pain (Campbell et al., 2018). The family environment is highly influential on thoughts and learning, with catastrophising and negative mood states also associated with dysfunctional EIH (Brellenthin et al., 2017). Family also provides a large source of social interactions where individuals may have been exposed to the notion that exercise can be harmful or pain should always be managed with rest and offloading. There may also be a physical contributor. If key family members are sedentary, this may lead to low activity levels among other family members. Social influences outside the family can also affect chronic pain (Martin, Tuttle & Mogil, 2014) and dysfunctional EIH. Uninformed vicarious learning can occur between peers and even from interactions with professionals. This form of 'social contagion' of misinformation can contribute to the failure of EIH mechanisms.

EIH responses may also be influenced by age, with older age groups showing a reduced EIH response to acute bouts of exercise compared to younger age groups; however, regular exercise may normalise the EIH response in older patients (Ohlman et al., 2018) and increased EIH has been shown in athletes when compared to normally active people (Tesarz et al., 2012). One potential mechanism for improved pain modulation may be that frequent physical activity increases opioid tone in the brainstem, which results in more nociceptive inhibition (Sluka et al., 2018).

Interestingly, there is an association between an individual's level of education and risk of persistent pain (Averill et al., 1996; Dahlhamer et al., 2018). Educational level is typically measured as a component of one's socio-economic status, the other components being income and occupation. It is important to note the potential for such a relationship to be reversed because persistent pain may also reduce socio-economic status.

In the same vein that there is a link between job autonomy and chronic pain (Teasell & Bombardier, 2001), there is also a link between exercise autonomy and effective EIH. Interesting animal research on mice showed that forced wheel running increased inflammation and mortality while voluntary wheel running had a protective effect (Cook et al., 2013). In another study, a positive effect on indicators of mood state, including antidepressive and anxiolytic (anti-anxiety) markers, were noted in mice completing voluntary wheel running (Duman et al., 2008). But how do humans respond to similar variables?

Lind, Ekkekakis and Vazou (2008) assessed a group of 25 middle-aged women participating in either self-paced treadmill exercises or increased pace running beyond the preferred exertion. The authors reported that even an increase of 10% above the preferred level led to a significant reduction in reported enjoyment, which could have a negative impact on adherence. One plausible link between these studies is the probability of increased psychological stress with forced exercise that may account for the more negative immune responses seen in mice. In Chapter 4, we look at how the nature of continuous low-level physical activity at work represents a similar involuntary activity environment.

This research indicates that the way we set exercises and the way individuals execute their rehabilitation programmes, including enjoyment and adherence factors, can be influential on their immune response and EIH. Perhaps, setting rigid exercise parameters is not favourable to exercise for pain relief, a concept that we discuss further in Chapter 7.

IMMUNE RESPONSES

Exercise-induced immune changes have been seen at local, central and systemic levels. The immune system responds to an acute bout of exercise and alters its response based on the frequency of the exercise stimulus. Regular physical activity promotes the release of more anti-inflammatory cytokines, whereas a lack of physical activity leads to the expression of more inflammatory cytokines (Sluka et al., 2018). In addition to inflammatory modulation, cytokines can also modulate nociceptive activity. At a more local level, exercising muscles release metabolites including macrophages. When comparing sedentary and regularly active people, there is a noted difference in the type of macrophages they release. Sedentary people release more M1 type macrophages, which release more inflammatory cytokines that stimulate local nociceptors. In contrast, more active people release M2 type macrophages, which release more anti-inflammatory cytokines that do not activate local nociceptors (Sluka et al., 2018).

MANAGING PATIENTS WITH DYSFUNCTIONAL EIH AND HYPERALGESIA

Imaging studies showed that brain regions involved with emotional, motivational and thought processes communicate directly with descending pain modulatory circuits (Ossipov, Morimura & Porreca, 2014). This is a two-way relationship as pain has also been shown to activate several brain areas, including sensory and emotional aspects. An appreciation of these influences and connections helps set the scene for the following discussion on how we can manage individuals with dysfunctional EIH.

EIH may be facilitated by some initial pain education to reduce the threat value of pain using cognitive behavioural and exposure therapy principles. As discussed at the start of this chapter, the aim is to educate the patient about the possibility of symptom flare-ups without creating a negative expectation nocebo effect.

As a general principle, pain during and after activity is acceptable but should dissipate quickly after stopping the exercise. If the opposite occurs and pain increases (a flare-up), then exercise intensity can be reduced. What should also occur is a reduced-pain flare-up with repeated bouts of exercise. I have experienced this in clinical practice. Such a pattern has been documented in the literature (Sandal et al., 2016) and it may occur for some of the reasons we have just discussed, including the immune response and increased opioid tone that occur as a patient shifts from sedentary to regular exercise. Undeniably, the pain experienced during this initial process is a major barrier to achieving a successful outcome.

Involving the patient in the planning process will create a patient-centred programme. The type of exercise used to trigger EIH need not be specific; therefore, patient preferences can be considered. Exercise should be easily achieved and enjoyable, which can be determined by the type of activity and whether it is completed at the client's preferred intensity.

Certain methods of encouraging EIH in the design of an exercise plan include avoiding eccentric and plyometric exercises because they are associated with delayed-onset muscle soreness.

Time contingents should be set up instead of ill-advising clients to stop if they feel pain. It can also be helpful to include multiple and long recovery breaks between exercise efforts. One reason individuals experience a negative outcome from exercise is that they do not allow enough time for adaptation and attempt to push themselves both within an individual session and over the course of the first few weeks. This is a common trigger for early rehabilitation pain flare-ups, which commonly dampen the individual's initial spark of motivation.

Another exercise phenomenon is the potential to reduce perceived pain from a joint by exercising a different joint (Lannersten & Kosek, 2010). A similar phenomenon occurs when you strengthen a muscle group on one side of the body and achieve improvements on the opposite side, known as the cross-education or cross-over effect; it has been suggested to aid rehabilitation by reducing atrophy in immobilised limbs during the early phases of recovery.

Dysfunctional EIH may be attenuated by combining centrally acting drugs with exercise. These could include opioids, serotonin and noradrenaline reuptake inhibitors, and selective serotonin reuptake inhibitors such as citalopram and sertraline (Nijs et al., 2012). These medications generally have a positive influence on mood state and pain and have been suggested to be supportive of EIH by stimulating otherwise absent or reduced descending inhibitory processes (Ossipov, Morimura & Porreca, 2014). Based on this approach, other analgesic treatments including manual therapy, and joint supports may be valuable additions to exercise; ideally, they should be applied just before or during exercise. These measures can then be reduced once routine and confidence have been established.

CONCLUSION

On recognising both the factors that influence EIH and the individuals less likely to experience it, an opportunity for pre-planning and client education exists to help aid the removal of any psychosocial barriers to EIH and communicate to clients the probable EIH outcomes based on their diagnosis.

We also need to balance positive outcome expectations with realistic ones; a realistic scenario may be the expectation of an after-exercise pain flare-up for an individual with fibromyalgia whereas a positive expectation would be the expected reductions in after-exercise flare-ups after routine sessions.

This chapter also presented ways to structure exercise programmes and activity to increase the probability of achieving successful EIH.

EIH provides a very non-specific approach to exercise for pain relief and is one of the key mechanisms by which exercise provides an analgesic response.

REFERENCES

Averill PM, Novy DM, Nelson DV, Berry LA (1996). Correlates of depression in chronic pain patients: a comprehensive examination. *Pain* 65:93–100.

Brellenthin AG, Crombie KM, Cook DB, Sehgal N, Koltyn KF (2017). Psychosocial influences on exercise-induced hypoalgesia. *Pain Med* 18:538–550.

Campbell P, Jordan KP, Smith BH, Generation Scotland, Dunn KM (2018). Chronic pain in families: a cross-sectional study of shared social, behavioural, and environmental influences. *Pain* 159:41–47.

Cook MD, Martin SA, Williams C, et al. (2013). Forced treadmill exercise training exacerbates inflammation and causes mortality while voluntary wheel training is protective in a mouse model of colitis. *Brain Behav Immun* 33:46–56.

Dahlhamer J, Lucas J, Zelaya C, et al. (2018). Prevalence of chronic pain and high-impact chronic pain among adults – United States, 2016. *MMWR Morb Mortal Wkly Rep* 67:1001–1006.

Duman CH, Schlesinger L, Russell DS, Duman RS (2008). Voluntary exercise produces antidepressant and anxiolytic behavioral effects in mice. *Brain Res* 1199:148–158.

Hoeger Bement MK, Dicapo J, Rasiarmos R, Hunter SK (2008). Dose response of isometric contractions on pain perception in healthy adults. *Med Sci Sports Exerc* 40:1880–1889.

Hoffmann P, Thorén P (1988). Electric muscle stimulation in the hind leg of the spontaneously hypertensive rat induces a long‐lasting fall in blood pressure. *Acta Physiol Scand* 133:211–219.

Koltyn KF (2002). Exercise-induced hypoalgesia and intensity of exercise. *Sports Med* 32:477–487.

Kosek E, Ekholm J, Hansson P (1996). Modulation of pressure pain thresholds during and following isometric contraction in patients with fibromyalgia and in healthy controls. *Pain* 64:415–423.

Lannersten L, Kosek E (2010). Dysfunction of endogenous pain inhibition during exercise with painful muscles in patients with shoulder myalgia and fibromyalgia. *Pain* 151:77–86.

Lind E, Ekkekakis P, Vazou S (2008). The affective impact of exercise intensity that slightly exceeds the preferred level. *J Health Psychol* 13:464–468.

Martin LJ, Tuttle AH, Mogil JS (2014). The interaction between pain and social behavior in humans and rodents. *Curr Top Behav Neurosci* 20:233–250.

Millan MJ (2002). Descending control of pain. *Prog Neurobiol* 66:355–474.

Naugle KM, Fillingim RB, Riley JL 3rd (2012). A meta-analytic review of the hypoalgesic effects of exercise. *J Pain* 13:1139–1150.

Nijs J, Kosek E, Van Oosterwijck J, Meeus M (2012). Dysfunctional endogenous analgesia during exercise in patients with chronic pain: to exercise or not to exercise? *Pain Physician* 15(3 Suppl):ES205–ES213.

Ohlman T, Miller L, Naugle KE, Naugle KM (2018). Physical activity levels predict exercise-induced hypoalgesia in older adults. *Med Sci Sports Exerc* 50:2101–2109.

Ossipov MH, Morimura K, Porreca F (2014). Descending pain modulation and chronification of pain. *Curr Opin Support Palliat Care* 8:143–151.

Racine M, Tousignant-Laflamme Y, Kloda LA, et al. (2012). A systematic literature review of 10 years of research on sex/gender and experimental pain perception – part 1: are there really differences between women and men? *Pain* 153:602–618.

Sandal LF, Roos EM, Bøgesvang SJ, Thorlund JB (2016). Pain trajectory and exercise-induced pain flares during 8 weeks of neuromuscular exercise in individuals with knee and hip pain. *Osteoarthritis Cartilage* 24:589–592.

Sluka KA, Frey-Law L, Bement MH (2018). Exercise-induced pain and analgesia? Underlying mechanisms and clinical translation. *Pain* 159:S91–S97.

Teasell RW, Bombardier C (2001). Employment-related factors in chronic pain and chronic pain disability. *Clin J Pain* 17(4 Supplement):S39–S45.

Tesarz J, Schuster AK, Hartmann M, Gerhardt A, Eich W (2012). Pain perception in athletes compared to normally active controls: a systematic review with meta-analysis. *Pain* 153:1253–1262.

Thorén P, Floras JS, Hoffmann P, Seals DR (1990). Endorphins and exercise: physiological mechanisms and clinical implications. *Med Sci Sports Exerc* 22:417–428.

Win R. *The Salt Path*. New York, NY: Penguin Books.

CHAPTER 4

THE PHYSICAL ACTIVITY PARADOX

INTRODUCTION

I would like to introduce you to the physical activity paradox; you are probably already aware of it, but perhaps not by this term. Have you ever questioned why some patients in active jobs are really unfit? Why that gardener you know who works physically all day has high blood pressure? Why that builder who is often lifting things at work has a bad back? Perhaps you know a farmer who is always active but suffers from chronic pain?

It is a widely accepted medical fact that physical activity is beneficial for our health, especially the cardiovascular system. In contrast, physical inactivity is a known risk factor for mortality, being ranked as fourth by the World Health Organization (2010), above obesity and below high blood glucose, both of which are also associated with inactivity. High blood pressure was ranked as the most prevalent risk factor.

In addition, many studies report the benefits of physical activity without specifying the context within which it is completed. For example, the World Health Organization stated in 2010 that in countries with high levels of occupational and transport physical activity, policymakers need to acknowledge that although these high levels of activity may not be the result of efforts to improve health, such levels of activity provide major health benefits for the population.

Despite this clear relationship between physical activity and reduced cardiovascular disease risk, the research indicates that there are significant differences between the risk reduction offered by leisure physical activity and the risk reduction offered by occupational physical activity. An article published in 2018 in the *British Journal of Sports Medicine* suggested why job-related physical activity differs from leisure physical activity (Holtermann et al., 2018).

I always thought there was a difference and this article clarified some of the factors I have been suspicious of in clinical practice.

This chapter identifies the proposed differences and underpinning mechanisms referencing additional research and clinical experiences. As always, I will strive to highlight the relevance of this information to the clinical setting.

LITERATURE REVIEW

Li, Loerbroks and Angerer (2013) reviewed 23 epidemiology studies published between 2011 and 2013. Their data analysis of over 790,000 adults found that moderate-to-high levels of leisure time physical activity were associated with reduced risk of coronary heart disease and stroke with a dose—response (more is better) relationship. When moderate-to-high levels were compared to low levels of leisure physical activity, the risk reduction range was 20–40%.

In contrast to leisure time activity, occupational activity showed an increased risk of cardiovascular disease within a 5–15% range for moderate levels of activity and an elevated risk range of 10–30% for high levels of occupational physical activity. These data suggest that occupational physical activity does not confer a similar protective effect on our health as leisure time physical activity. In fact, Holtermann et al. (2018) go as far as to suggest that occupational and leisure-based physical activity may have opposing effects on health. This may be due to many factors including the volume of physical activity. One study of active commuting (on foot or bicycle) and leisure time physical activity found a reduction in cardiovascular disease risk unless physical activity exceeded 60 minutes, whereupon such volume was associated with increased resting blood pressure measurements (Hu et al., 2002).

Physical activity at work typically lasts for many hours with repetitive tasks and prolonged static postures that can cause elevated blood pressure, which, if sustained over long periods of time, can be a risk factor for cardiovascular disease (Mancia et al., 2017).

The lack of ability to choose tasks, adjust work rate, take rest breaks and a general lack of autonomy may also increase psychological stress. This is similar to the identified different outcomes between forced and voluntary exercise we discussed in Chapter 3. Murine studies reported adverse immune responses for forced exercise (Cook et al., 2013), while a human study reported reduced enjoyment with forced exercise intensity (Lind, Ekkekakis & Vazou, 2008).

Furthermore, job-related physical activity is often too low in intensity to increase cardiovascular health or musculoskeletal strength. This identified insufficient exercise stimulus may lead to poor health if a stimulus is not provided outside of work. Individuals may make the incorrect assumption that they are meeting their exercise targets within the working day. In addition, the energy cost of their job may also reduce motivation to take leisure exercise. I see this a lot in the clinic when people have a physical job coupled with family responsibilities. Some people really do or would struggle to meet national exercise guidelines.

Some of the benefits of physical activity may result from its effect on inflammatory processes; the body responds to an acute bout of exercise with increased inflammatory mediators matched with protective anti-inflammatory processes. Regular physical activity reduces resting inflammatory mediator levels via multiple suggested mechanisms, including a decrease in adipose tissue-initiated inflammation and skeletal muscle-initiated inflammation (Kasapis & Thompson, 2005). However, without a defined stimulus–response–rest–adaptation pattern and with more continued physical activity exposure, inflammatory markers may remain elevated for prolonged periods of time and this has been associated with increased cardiovascular disease risk. The proposed inflammatory contribution to atherosclerosis (Ross, 1999) may provide a mechanistic link for this increased cardiovascular disease risk.

Mechanistically, this health paradox may in part be explained by the different effects of occupational versus leisure activity on the autonomic nervous system. The potential for continued stress caused by occupational physical activity can lead to dysregulation of the autonomic nervous system by creating an imbalance in the sympathetic and parasympathetic drives (Thayer & Lane, 2007). This imbalanced autonomic regulation is associated with increased cardiovascular disease risk (Thayer, Yamamoto & Brosschot, 2010), the causes of which may be reduced baroreceptor activity from increased vascular stiffness and reduced heart rate variability, endothelial dysfunction associated with all major cardiovascular risk factors (Joyner & Green, 2009), elevated blood pressure and excess proinflammatory cytokines (Tracey, 2002).

CONCLUSION

When enquiring about activity levels, if a patient mentions something like 'I keep fit at work', we now know that research questions the efficacy of occupational physical activity being classed as therapeutic exercise or its ability to offer a sufficient stimulus. It also has the potential to be the cause of poor health.

Occupational activity needs to be understood and factored into the individual's exercise plan; it is different than leisure activity but it may still influence their overall stress and recovery.

In fact, long working hours completing physical tasks may provide a comparable mechanism to that seen in overtraining syndrome in endurance athletes, where too much training stimulus is paired with insufficient recovery time. In an occupational setting, physical activity intensity may be lower but last for longer than athletic endurance training; furthermore, recovery periods may be lacking. As already mentioned, the combination of leisure physical activity coupled with high occupational physical activities may create an increased risk of overtraining syndrome. Also, the benefits of leisure time physical activity may be reduced or even reversed if coupled with high levels of occupational physical activity; again, the overall lack of recovery may cause an autonomic imbalance (Hallman et al., 2017).

Research supports specific leisure activity as superior to and different from work-related physical activity. There is a risk of misinterpreting this evidence to suggest that exercise at work is bad for you! This would be a gross oversimplification, but the physical activity paradox clarifies that the difference between job-related activity and leisure activity is significant enough to factor it into our assessment and rehabilitation planning.

REFERENCES

Cook MD, Martin SA, Williams C, et al. (2013). Forced treadmill exercise training exacerbates inflammation and causes mortality while voluntary wheel training is protective in a mouse model of colitis. *Brain Behav Immun* 33:46–56.

Holtermann A, Krause N, van der Beek AJ, Straker L (2018). The physical activity paradox: six reasons why occupational physical activity (OPA) does not confer the cardiovascular health benefits that leisure time physical activity does. *Br J Sports Med* 52:149–150.

Hu G, Pekkarinen H, Hänninen O, et al. (2002). Commuting, leisure-time physical activity, and cardiovascular risk factors in China. *Med Sci Sports Exerc* 34:234–238.

Joyner MJ, Green DJ (2009). Exercise protects the cardiovascular system: effects beyond traditional risk factors. *J Physiol* 587:5551–5558.

Kasapis C, Thompson PD (2005). The effects of physical activity on serum C-reactive protein and inflammatory markers: a systematic review. *J Am Coll Cardiol* 45:1563–1569.

Li J, Loerbroks A, Angerer P (2013). Physical activity and risk of cardiovascular disease: what does the new epidemiological evidence show? *Curr Opin Cardiol* 28:575–583.

Lind E, Ekkekakis P, Vazou S (2008). The affective impact of exercise intensity that slightly exceeds the preferred level: 'pain' for no additional 'gain'. *J Health Psychol* 13:464–468.

Mancia G, Bombelli M, Cuspidi C, Facchetti R, Grassi G (2017). Cardiovascular risk associated with white-coat hypertension response to increased cardiovascular risk of white-coat hypertension: pro side of the argument. *Hypertension* 70:668–675.

Ross R (1999). Atherosclerosis—an inflammatory disease. *N Engl J Med* 340:115–126.

Thayer JF, Lane RD (2007). The role of vagal function in the risk for cardiovascular disease and mortality. *Biol Psychol* 74:224–242.

Thayer JF, Yamamoto SS, Brosschot JF (2010). The relationship of autonomic imbalance, heart rate variability and cardiovascular disease risk factors. *Int J Cardiol* 141:122–131.

Tracey KJ (2002). The inflammatory reflex. *Nature* 420:853–859.

World Health Organization (2010). *Global Recommendations on Physical Activity for Health*. Geneva: World Health Organization. Available at https://www.who.int/publications/i/item/9789241599979 (accessed 18 June 2023).

CHAPTER 5

PLACEBO OR NOCEBO: PREPARING TO EXERCISE

INTRODUCTION

From my experience as both physiotherapist and educator, the term placebo is perhaps one of the most misunderstood terms in health care. Many people consider a placebo to be a negative thing. Placebos are not negative and are often a powerful part of treatment and recovery.

Perhaps one of the reasons why the placebo effect might be viewed negatively is the suggestion that it is a form of deception. When an individual believes they are receiving an active treatment but are in fact receiving an inactive treatment, this could be considered a form of deception and creates ethical barriers in research design, barriers that hinder the progression of health care and ironically often sustain poor or deceptive practices. It is more complex when the patient receives the active treatment but the associated positive outcome is caused by the placebo effect and not the active treatment itself. The positive outcome is often attributed to the intervention; when compared to a different or no intervention, the results favour the intervention. It is only when you compare the intervention to a sham treatment and successfully blind participants to whether they are receiving the real or sham intervention that you can start to see if it is the intervention itself or just a placebo effect.

That is why comparing surgery to exercise in research studies does not prove or disprove the efficacy of surgery because both groups would have very different experiences of treatment. As you can imagine, the surgical group would be much more expectant of rapid results after an objective procedure whereas exercise groups are often left feeling underwhelmed and undertreated.

I hope you can now begin to appreciate that the placebo effect is multifactorial and would therefore also form a component of any active treatment. We will also discover that outcome expectancy can alter the outcome of both active and inert treatments.

Prising the placebo from active elements is one of the great challenges of research trials.

Although much of the placebo research has been done in pharmacology, we can turn our attention to the placebo effect in physical therapies and consider some of the available research.

I have certainly shocked many students when I tell them that much of what a manual therapist achieves is due to a placebo effect. For the record, I am a keen manual therapist. When I tell students that some common surgeries are mainly placebo, they are often resistant to any such idea. Of course, this does not refer to all surgery and I will justify my statement by highlighting some of the surgical research that compares active surgery to sham surgery for musculoskeletal conditions such as subacromial impingement syndrome (Beard et al., 2018) or meniscal tears (Sihvonen et al., 2013). We will return to this research again to review it in more detail.

Historically, the placebo effect has been theoretical and hard to define but now, due to modern imaging methods, we know that the placebo effect is a real neurobiological phenomenon that mediates psychobiological and behavioural changes vital to healing processes. We now have a better understanding of this phenomenon that includes positive outcome expectation and, for the more spiritual reader, faith in recovery.

The placebo effect is not defined as a specific effect and it is very variable. The placebo effect also covers many different types of input and is not a single entity. It is very much an umbrella term that needs dismantling if we are to understand its influences in a way that allows us to shape our treatment outcomes.

In research, a placebo is usually an inert pill that is presented as an active drug. This is the reason why placebos are often considered by the general public to be a physical entity. However, placebos can come in many forms, such as word interpretation, ritualistic behaviour, image associations and positive expectation, all of which act centrally on the higher centres of the brain; this helps the brain contextualise input and determine our body's multi-system responses.

THE NOCEBO EFFECT

This chapter would not be complete without introducing the opposite to the placebo effect, that is, the nocebo effect.

A nocebo is defined as a harmless entity, thought or feeling that when experienced is associated with harmful effects due to negative expectations or associations. I can provide a couple of simple examples. Telling a patient that a specific exercise will make their knee pain much worse would be a nocebo. Showing a patient a gory image of a degenerative joint and suggesting that this relates to their joint will probably increase their pain perception and produce a significant nocebo stimulus.

In our dealings with patients, while some of our communications will be neutral, it is probable that most of what we do or say will have either a nocebo or placebo influence, so it is in our interests to learn more to enhance our patient outcomes.

HOW DOES THE PLACEBO EFFECT WORK?

One of the key mechanisms for placebo analgesia is the stimulation of endogenous opioids and descending inhibitory mechanisms. This links our discussion on exercise-induced hypoalgesia in Chapter 3 to the importance of the placebo effect in the analgesic response to exercise. The expectation of pain relief activates opioid receptor signalling in the brain (Zubieta et al., 2005) with identified responses in brain structures associated with pain modulation and in pivotal areas of the descending pain control system (Eippert et al., 2009). The placebo effect covers more than just analgesia; it also stimulates the immune system and specifically mediates the inflammatory response. The widespread mechanisms of the placebo effect provide a biological basis for the power of thought and the self-healing capabilities of the body.

WHAT FACTORS INFLUENCE THE PLACEBO OR NOCEBO EFFECT?

Suggestion and expectancy have been recognised as key instigators of the placebo or nocebo reaction (Colloca & Miller, 2011). A classical conditioning Pavlovian theory is also supported by pharmacology research where the benefits of taking a routine active medication are identified to continue even after the medication is switched to an inactive ingredient, most commonly a sugar pill (Tekampe et al., 2018).

The aforementioned example supports the theory that the placebo effect is a learning phenomenon whereby previous experience of a therapeutic outcome has an important role; successful repetition of an effective outcome makes the placebo effect more robust in the face of future exposures. Therapeutic experience has an important role in the responsiveness of placebos.

Family and social interactions can cause a placebo or nocebo response. In many cultures, older family members are traditionally consulted for advice and their knowledge is often afforded more credibility than advice from medically qualified individuals. Advice from less credible sources can also gain a foothold of conscious consideration through repetition; if you hear something frequently enough, you are increasingly likely to believe it. This can occur through regular contact with social groups who hold certain health beliefs or from repetitive health care adverts popping up on your social media feeds.

Unfortunately, placebo and nocebo learning is unbalanced and more heavily weighted in favour of the nocebo effect, which appears to take less conditioning in the form of repetition of associations (Colloca & Benedetti, 2006). It has been suggested that a nocebo effect can be set up simply by verbal suggestion whereas a placebo effect of equal magnitude would require a first-hand experience of a positive outcome to cause an effective placebo conditioning procedure (Colloca, Sigaudo & Benedetti, 2008). Therefore, whereas learning is less critical for nocebo responses, it is fundamental in placebo responses (Colloca & Benedetti, 2006; Colloca, Sigaudo & Benedetti, 2008).

An example of a placebo conditioning procedure would be an individual experiencing pain relief after physical activity. This experience could be enhanced by explaining to the individual the theory of exercise-induced hypoalgesia both before and after physical activity. This would serve to strengthen a placebo effect by increasing the expectancy of a positive outcome. Even after a conditioning procedure, expectation has a key role. Expectations are mediators of outcome.

While I personally do not feel suitably informed to write about spiritual influences and ritualistic behaviours, these are factors that have been identified to trigger a placebo effect. Green (2006) provided an eloquent review of the pre-treatment ritualistic similarities between surgeons and shamans. A surgeon himself, he identified the important contribution of patient suggestibility and thus the placebo effect. From an academic standpoint, there may be similarities between ritual theory and placebo theory. For further reading, I recommend *Surgery, the Ultimate Placebo* by orthopaedic surgeon Ian Harris (2016).

PLACEBO EXAMPLES AND MORAL CONUNDRUMS

In musculoskeletal medicine, one of the most common supplements I am often asked about is glucosamine. I hold the following knowledge regarding this supplement in my memory to share with clients.

A review of independent and supplement industry-funded trials assessing the effects of glucosamine or chondroitin supplements on joint pain and radiological progression of disease in patients with osteoarthritis of the hip or knee identified that chondroitin or glucosamine alone or combined did not have a clinically relevant effect on perceived joint pain or on joint space narrowing. The authors stated that these supplements are not harmful and can be given to patients as long as patients perceive a benefit and pay for their own treatment (Wandel et al., 2010). So the health care provider is not paying for ineffective treatment but the patient can pay to benefit from the placebo effect. Is it not the moral duty of the professional to share the research results and offer the client the chance to avoid wasting money? Here is another example.

Here is another example. I meet many clients who are waiting for subacromial decompression surgery. This is now generally considered an ineffective surgery after research, including a study by Beard et al (2018), identified that it is no better than sham surgery. I have heard some doctors suggest that the procedure can still be justified even on the basis of a placebo effect. The unnecessary cost and health risks of surgery make this a hollow argument. Having placebo surgery is not akin to placebo supplements or manual therapies. The costs, resources and risks are not negligible—they are very significant.

A NOCEBO EXAMPLE

Negative expectancy has the power to potentially neutralise treatments with known effectiveness. This phenomenon was reported in a pharmacological study showing that negative expectancy neutralised the pain-relieving effect of a potent opioid medication at both a behavioural and neural level (Bingel et al., 2011). In the study, healthy volunteers were administered a fixed concentration of a powerful pain relief medication called remifentanil and exposed to a painful heat stimulus. They were then assessed under three different conditions: expecting pain relief; not expecting pain relief; and expecting an increase in pain.

When the volunteers expected pain relief, the analgesic effect of the medications was doubled. In contrast, when the volunteers expected the pain to increase, the analgesic effect of the medication was neutralised.

If the expectation of an increase in pain had led to a doubling of pain perception, this would have shown that the medication was inactive and only a placebo.

Remifentanil is a powerful analgesic opioid but this study highlights that its efficacy is heavily influenced by a placebo or nocebo effect. We can extrapolate these results and consider how our own manual therapy and exercise interventions could be more informed by expectations than we have previously considered.

A JOURNEY OF MANY PLACEBOS

As I mentioned earlier, the increased attention afforded to the placebo effect is not new. Placebos and nocebos are natural occurrences that have been identified, labelled and researched to gain a better understanding of how they could be used to enhance treatment outcomes.

Let us consider a typical patient journey from first deciding that they need some treatment to actually receiving it and identify a few likely incidences where a placebo or nocebo could take effect.

On identifying that they need treatment, an individual will probably seek a recommendation from a friend. A positive recommendation is the first exposure to a placebo effect that triggers a positive outcome expectation. If the individual then has a positive or at least neutral experience of arranging an appointment with you, then this carries the placebo effect through to when they first arrive at your clinic; this is perhaps the first time that images or physical factors can exert their placebo effect. Simple things such as how easy the parking is. The location of your clinic. The overall appearance. How your front door looks. How easy it is to access the building and then the inside of the building, including the receptionist and the ambiance in the waiting room. All of these provide a placebo (or nocebo) effect.

Initial interactions with anybody within your clinic (not just your reception team), other members of staff, other patients and of course finally you, can be highly impactful on the placebo effect. This is all before you have even conversed with your client.

There are also much more subtle influences such as the colour of your walls, the smell in your clinic and maybe your smell too. There are then the much more tangible interactions such as any therapeutic tools that you may use, from ultrasound machines to vibrating massage tools; these all carry with them the potential for a powerful placebo effect and of course all of these extrinsic things are filtered and interpreted by our clients' intrinsic experiences and belief systems. One clinical example from my experience is spinal manipulation; some individuals feel better just knowing that you are going to 'click' their spine while others may immediately feel more pain just thinking about it. The same technique can offer a placebo for one person and a nocebo for another.

CLINICAL STRATEGIES TO MANAGE THE PLACEBO AND NOCEBO EFFECTS

When it comes to the communication between you and your patient, significant research has been done on the importance of the words that we use and the influences that these can have on individuals' thoughts, feelings and levels of anxiety. If pills are the main source of placebo in medicine and procedures are the main source of placebo in surgery, then in physical therapy it may be our use of language and the words we use or choose to consciously avoid. Of course, we also have clinical tools and treatment procedures, but the use of language is receiving the most attention in the literature and filling more lecture slots at conferences.

THE IMPACT OF COMMUNICATION

Our words and attitudes towards our clients can induce immediate worsening of symptom severity. I expect you can easily conjure up a scene in your head of a glum therapist explaining a diagnosis in the most dour way, but clients can also suffer in the presence of the most positive and enthusiastic clinician if there is a mismatch in mood and expectancy. Imagine if your back felt 'locked' in a painful spasm and you were anxious about movement. The last thing you would want is a manual therapist pulling and yanking you around in an overzealous manner!

One of the biggest non-physical challenges I have is trying to clear clients' previous misconceptions of their pain. Previous information sources may have been wrong or misinterpreted and seemingly harmless medical terms can mean different things to our clients.

A balance must exist between communicating important clinical findings in a non-deceptive, honest way while minimising the negative nocebo effect of the communication.

In an interesting qualitative study, Barker, Reid and Minns Lowe (2009) asked members of the public for their interpretations of common terms used when receiving back pain treatment from either a chiropractor, osteopath or physiotherapist. The terms were then categorised into three groups:

1. Terms that could lead to problematic misunderstandings, for example, chronic, instability, neurological involvement, wear and tear, arthritis.

2. Terms with unintended meanings but few negative repercussions, for example, mechanical back pain, sciatica, muscle imbalance, prolapsed disc, alignment.
3. Terms that the public appeared to understand as intended, for example, muscle spasm, manipulation, soft-tissue technique, rehabilitation.

Problematic words are not all 'wrong' in their usage, only in their interpretation, and not everyone will interpret them incorrectly. My personal interpretation of the research is that I now take more time to explain and ask the client to clarify their understanding during consultations. I am also much more careful with the word 'instability' now, not letting it wobble around my conversations.

So once the client is with you in person or on the phone, they are susceptible to your influence on their pain experience. It is important to realise that we need to pay attention to what we say, choosing our words carefully because words themselves are treatments. We can use a positive phrase like 'your hip has good range of movement and has the potential to be stronger and to support the joint more' or a negative phrase like 'your hip is unstable because you have muscle atrophy'.

COMMUNICATING X-RAY RESULTS

X-rays often form part of my clients' assessments; reporting the results in the context of how the images relate to the presenting symptoms is important. I typically do a few things to reduce the threat value of these results. First, I check the relevance of the result: Is it the correct limb? Correct joint? Correct tissue? Next, I attempt to put the report in context. If the report states 'loss of joint space', you cannot say 'oh it's all fine'; that would be a lie and could get you in trouble for either lying or not being able to read! Instead I would say, 'the X-ray reports some typical age-related changes and notes some narrowing of the joint space on one side of your knee; this is a typical finding and is probably found in lots of peoples' knees. It is also important to note that it is possibly not the cause of the pain.

From this point, I then help them build a real appreciation for what a real joint actually is; it is certainly not a few bones and ligaments like most plastic anatomy models shown in the clinic. Joints are a complex system of contractile and non-contractile tissues that dissipate and produce forces during movement, with intricate multi-level control from the brain and nervous system. The next time you reach for the plastic joint to explain a diagnosis, just stop and think whether it will help or hinder your patient.

SOME QUICK-FIRE TIPS FOR THE CLINIC

Managing expectations

- Optimise positive expectations while being realistic and evidence-based where possible.
- Manage expectations from the start to avoid an expectation mismatch.
- Raise awareness of potential adverse effects, normalise them and discuss management strategies. No surprises!
- Teach coping strategies for flare-ups.
- Show helpful information sources like websites.

- Use observational learning videos and patient success examples.
- Advocate suitable patient support groups.

Communication

- Listen first.
- Understand, care and show empathy.
- Provide contextual information on assessment and treatment options.
- Ask questions to understand your client's perspective and reduce misunderstandings.
- Assess clients' thoughts, behaviours and expectations.
- Medical jargon is likely to cause misunderstandings (unless they are a medical professional).

CONCLUSION

If the placebo effect is powerful enough, we can question the very efficacy of any active treatment intervention and appreciate how the associated placebo elements may in fact summate to be the primary driver of a positive outcome. I appreciate that this is a very bold statement to make and one that might imply that I am suggesting that all we do as physical therapists is create a placebo effect. However, I am biased by the topic of this chapter and my opinions are informed by research into this area that populates many divisions of health care research. While many readers may continue to feel uncomfortable openly suggesting that the placebo effect largely influences your work as a practitioner, and I appreciate that telling your clients 'to have faith' is just not going to happen within your four walls of evidenced-based practice, I must point out that the similar term 'outcome expectation' emerges with increasing frequency in persistent pain research. Are they not the same thing?

The success of even the best evidence-based exercise we dream up is determined by the client's willingness to complete it and their appreciation of its chances of success.

Doubts, concerns, misunderstandings, miscommunications and a lack of information will create barriers to rehabilitation; this is really important because if an individual does not believe and understand the rehabilitation plan, then the plan will not work.

I hope that you were already aware of some of the concepts presented in this chapter. I hope you also found some new insights to help improve your practice. If I also challenged your current beliefs and made you feel a little uncomfortable, then I will have achieved the main aim of the chapter. A book full of things you already know is a pointless read, a book of teaching that you agree with is of limited value, whereas a book that challenges our beliefs offers the greatest potential for learning. Afterall, we learn more from someone who challenges our beliefs than from someone who agrees with them. *Would you agree?*

REFERENCES

Barker KL, Reid M, Minns Lowe CJ (2009). Divided by a lack of common language? A qualitative study exploring the use of language by health professionals treating back pain. *BMC Musculoskelet Disord* 10:123.

Beard DJ, Rees JL, Cook JA, et al. (2018). Arthroscopic subacromial decompression for subacromial shoulder pain (CSAW): a multicentre, pragmatic, parallel group, placebo-controlled, three-group, randomised surgical trial. *Lancet* 391:329–338.

Bingel U, Wanigasekera V, Wiech K, et al. (2011) The effect of treatment expectation on drug efficacy: imaging the analgesic benefit of the opioid remifentanil. *Sci Transl Med* 3:70ra14.

Colloca L, Benedetti F (2006). How prior experience shapes placebo analgesia. *Pain* 124:126–133.

Colloca L, Miller FG (2011). How placebo responses are formed: a learning perspective. *Philos Trans R Soc Lond B Biol Sci* 366:1859–1869.

Colloca L, Sigaudo M, Benedetti F (2008). The role of learning in nocebo and placebo effects. *Pain* 136:211–218.

Eippert F, Bingel U, Schoell ED, et al. (2009). Activation of the opioidergic descending pain control system underlies placebo analgesia. *Neuron* 63:533–543.

Green SA (2006). Surgeons and shamans. *Clin Orthop Relat Res* 450:249–254.

Harris I (2016). *Surgery, the Ultimate Placebo: a Surgeon Cuts Through the Evidence*. Sydney, NSW: UNSW Press.

Sihvonen R, Paavola M, Malmivaara A, et al. (2013). Arthroscopic partial meniscectomy versus sham surgery for a degenerative meniscal tear. *N Engl J Med* 369:2515–2524.

Tekampe J, van Middendorp H, Sweep FCGJ, et al. (2018). Human pharmacological conditioning of the immune and endocrine system: challenges and opportunities. *Int Rev Neurobiol* 138:61–80.

Wandel S, Jüni P, Tendal B, et al. (2010). Effects of glucosamine, chondroitin, or placebo in patients with osteoarthritis of hip or knee: network meta-analysis. *BMJ* 341:c4675.

Zubieta J-K, Bueller JA, Jackson LR, et al. (2005). Placebo effects mediated by endogenous opioid activity on mu-opioid receptors. *J Neurosci* 25:7754–7762.

BIBLIOGRAPHY

Hyland ME (2011). Motivation and placebos: do different mechanisms occur in different contexts? *Philos Trans R Soc Lond B Biol Sci* 366:1828–1837.

Meissner K, Kohls N, Colloca L (2011). Introduction to placebo effects in medicine: mechanisms and clinical implications. *Philos Trans R Soc Lond B Biol Sci* 366:1783–1789.

Pollo A, Carlino E, Benedetti F (2011). Placebo mechanisms across different conditions: from the clinical setting to physical performance. *Philos Trans R Soc Lond B Biol Sci* 366:1790–1798.

CHAPTER 6

PAIN EDUCATION, COGNITIVE BEHAVIOURAL THERAPY AND MOTIVATIONAL INTERVIEWING

INTRODUCTION

A deeper understanding of the impact our thoughts have on exercise behaviours would empower physical rehabilitators with a vital core skill. We also need to appreciate that unless you are a trained and experienced psychotherapist, you should always be aware of practising inside your professional scope and skill set. There is always the potential to trigger a patient response that you do not have the skill to deal with. This requires the measured incorporation of cognition management into exercise rehabilitation.

In this chapter, I introduce pain education, cognitive behavioural therapy and motivational interviewing. You may have heard about, or already use, these well-known and researched approaches; if not, I am sure you will find them as useful as I do. I have carefully selected their inclusion based on evidence from the literature and success in my own clinic.

This chapter is one of the book's most important ones because the impact of cognition on exercise outcome, physical function and pain relief is often overlooked and under-represented in many education programmes, often in favour of teaching special tests and more formal treatment modalities. This is changing, but from my observations and from speaking with students it remains the norm in many institutions.

Every time a well-intentioned prescribed rehabilitation exercise fails to reduce pain, we are potentially reinforcing the negative expectation for that individual and increasing the risk of losing another client, who may then seek less effective and potentially detrimental treatments. For this reason, it is in our best interests to reduce these negative outcomes as much as possible and promote the efficacy of exercise for pain relief and the publicly perceived value of our profession.

To keep a sense of perspective, my experience has taught me, and the evidence informs us, that there is a success rate for physical rehabilitation for pain relief and this success rate varies widely depending on ailment, joint and the treatment technique used. For example, there is no such thing as a 100% success rate for back, neck and shoulder pain treatments. Gurus do not exist and people who write books about pain do not cure all of their clients of pain, myself included. So, if you find yourself frustrated by a client's lack of recovery, rest assured that you are not alone in your experience. In reality, all health care professionals struggle to help certain clients and some clients are very difficult to help. We are all on a mission to help our clients and improve our skills. After reading this chapter, you will improve your clients' outcomes but you will still not reach the mythical 100% success rate. Do not let this frustrate you; instead, let it motivate you to keep reading and keep learning.

COGNITIVE BEHAVIOURAL THERAPY

In this section, we are going to work with the thoughts, behaviours and emotions clients share with us during consultations. We do this with a background knowledge of the three core tenets of cognitive behavioural therapy (CBT).

When we understand a client's thoughts, behaviours and emotions, we can begin to analyse and evaluate them using CBT to identify and break down barriers to exercise and recovery.

CBT is based on the combination of basic principles from behavioural and cognitive psychology. CBT is described and used in different ways. In this chapter, I use a few useful CBT principles that you can easily apply to exercise rehabilitation.

While the formalised ideas of cognitive therapy and CBT have only been around for 30–40 years, the very notion that people's perceptions of events is the key determinant of their experience is an ancient one, as demonstrated by Epictetus (**Figure 6.1**).

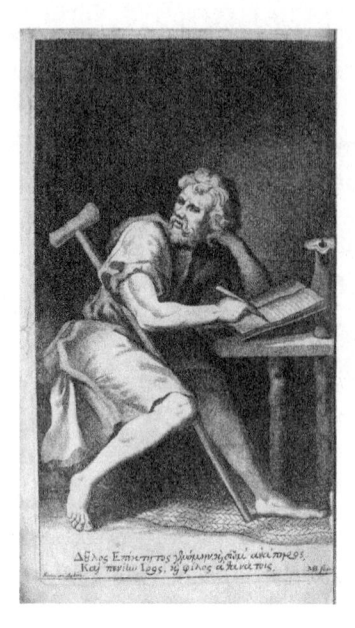

Figure 6.1: 'People are disturbed not by events alone but by the views they take of them (Epictetus 55–135 AD)'. Engraved frontispiece of Edward Ivie's Latin translation (or versification) of Epictetus' *Enchiridon*, printed in Oxford in 1715. *Source*: William Sonmans, public domain via Wikimedia Commons.

The components of CBT are shown in Figure 6.2 to represent their interrelated influence; they are not stand-alone entities.

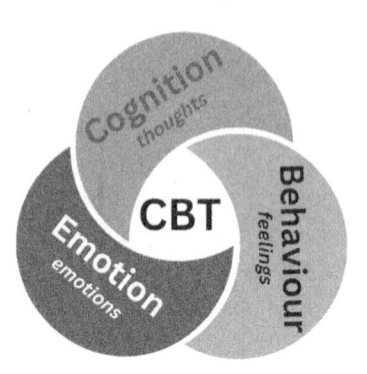

Figure 6.2: The three categories of patient information we are interested in with CBT.

You can use a simple form like the one shown in Table 6.1 to unassumingly capture the client's thoughts, behaviours and emotions. More direct questioning may be necessary with reserved clients but I try to pick out the required information through relaxed conversation that focuses more on listening than questioning.

Table 6.1: CBT examples

COGNITION (THOUGHTS)	BEHAVIOUR (ACTIONS)	EMOTION (FEELINGS)
Pain means that damage is occurring.	Not putting any weight through a painful joint.	Anxiety about what is really going on inside my body.
This knee pain is because running is bad for my knees.	Taking it easy and discouraging my children from running.	Frustrated I did not know before and worry my children might do the same.
I will have to stop work because this job is bad for my back.	Looking for a sitting-based office job.	Sadness over a planned job change.
I need to start looking after myself better.	Looking for a walking group or a gym.	Positive but anxious about planned changes.
Arthritis means the joint is crumbling.	Continuously nursing the joint even when inactive.	Anxiety and fear of further pain and harm.

Abbreviation: CBT, cognitive behavioural therapy.

A strong relationship with the client is a vital determinant of CBT success and overall behavioural change. The building of a working relationship takes time and is strengthened over time, so make sure you allow your assessments to continue over multiple sessions and not limit them to one initial assessment. This is a mistake I made too many times early in my career. My first client contact was always a time-limited initial assessment with the aim of stating a diagnosis to satisfy them. Subsequent sessions were then termed treatment sessions. My advice to you is, let the assessment continue.

Based on the content of this chapter, I would encourage you to keep assessing and getting to know what your clients think, do and feel during subsequent follow-up sessions. This strategy will help you unearth those invisible barriers to a successful rehabilitation outcome.

I should also note that cognitive therapies for pain are challenged by the pain itself. Pain is an emotional experience that interferes with cognitive functioning, making it more difficult to rationalise the pain. Therefore, clients in pain are often more resistant to new information from health care providers or just less able to process it.

EDUCATING PATIENTS ABOUT PAIN

When we review our clients' thoughts, behaviours and emotions, they are mostly responses to pain or fear of pain. Therefore, if they (or we) cannot eliminate their pain, as we experience with so many clients, it then commonly becomes their maladaptive response to pain that requires understanding and change. This relates to both acute pain from strains and sprains and more complex persistent (chronic) pain. It is important to remember that the response to recent-onset pain can sometimes determine longer-term pain processing changes. Education about pain is much more central in complex pain clients but, in many cases, pain knowledge may serve a protective function by preventing more complex changes from developing in the first instance.

An irrational fear of movement due to pain (kinesiophobia) makes individuals hypervigilant, tuning into every change in body sensation, every ache and niggle and, as a result, often responding with increased muscle tension and movement restriction. Cognitive processes (thoughts) are hugely influential to pain perception. For example, an individual with chest pain who thinks it may be a heart attack is going to respond to the pain in a very different way to an individual experiencing pain in their wrist without a previous injury. One is frustrating (wrist pain), the other is potentially fatal (chest pain). Thus, because pain lacks an external reference, it is highly dependent on personal interpretation.

Pain education is also an important part of our own professional education and an important part of the therapist–client interaction.

If we are being honest with ourselves as professionals, we might acknowledge that educating clients about pain is difficult and often fails. From my experience and research, I believe this is for two fundamental reasons: (1) the client resists any change to their current, often biomedical, ideas of pain, possibly because they feel that structural theories help to validate their pain among health care professionals whose empathy often wanes over time; and (2) the misunderstanding that a professional is now telling them that 'it is all in their head' and the incorrect notion that a physical issue is now a psychological one.

CATASTROPHISING

Catastrophising is a key determinant of an individual's ability to manage pain. It can cause changes to the brain's sensory processing and increase the likelihood of a pain response. You will often hear your clients expressing catastrophic misinterpretations of bodily sensations with comments like: my back has gone; this hip is completely shot; I can feel my knee is bone on bone; I feel this pain is something serious. In contrast, there is also a patient population whose symptom reporting is so minimal they often ignore signs and symptoms that are serious. While this is not the population we typically meet in our clinics, it serves to remind us of the importance of getting to know the client and not just their symptoms and of the fact that pain is present for a reason; in some circumstances, the pain may be trying to send an important message.

It is important to state that kinesiophobia and catastrophising are really very normal reactions that routinely occur with varied intensity in the general population. I am sure you can think of some examples of when you limited your own movement or panicked over a small physical niggle. We need to recognise the normality of these reactions and not be too quick to label them as psychological pathologies. The aim is to treat the individual, not the diagnosis.

EXPLAINING PAIN

So how do I explain pain to my clients? I struggled repeatedly to get a coherent and consistent message across, so I wrote down my explanation and recorded it in a video hosted on my YouTube Channel—The Physio Channel (How to explain pain to a patient; https://youtu.be/Zsoo-EcxD3A).

The video transcript is as follows…

If you are in pain, it is a horrible experience. It is only natural to want to know what is causing it. Perhaps you have already been told the cause by your doctor or given different answers from other professionals leading you to become confused. It is also likely that you have tried to tackle the cause of the pain but the pain has persisted or returned, again causing confusion regarding the source of the pain.

This is a video for people suffering from pain who want to have a better understanding of why. In this video I explain what pain is and what it is not.

Pain is always real and pain is not all in your mind. This is the most common misunderstanding when medical professionals try to explain pain to patients.

Research has taught us much about pain over the last 20 years. Some people, including professionals, still use traditional assessment and treatment methods that are now scientifically outdated. I produced this video to help you have a more informed understanding of your pain.

The good news is that just learning about and understanding your pain can reduce it. This is because a greater understanding of the pain experience and how to manage it can reduce worry, anxiety and stress, all of which are powerful influencers of pain severity.

'Pain' is a single word that can mean so many different things, from a niggling ache to excruciatingly stabbing. It is nearly always an unpleasant sensation with an emotional attachment.

As I mentioned already, pain is always real but because you cannot see it on a scan or remove it surgically, there is an often unspoken void between you and the person assessing your pain. They are reliant on your explanation. You may have felt that your doctor or therapist did not fully understand your pain. The two great challenges of pain assessment are determining its source and understanding what it means to you as a patient and as an individual; thus, expressing your feelings about the pain you are experiencing can be much more helpful than saying it is a 7 out of 10 or an 11 out of 10. This is because your thoughts and feelings can have a significant impact on your pain. I will explain this in more depth.

I mentioned at the start of the video that the notion that pain is all in your head is incorrect. Let us have a look at what is correct with an outline of our historical and then current understanding of pain, without using too much medical jargon.

The old model of pain (as exemplified by the pain pathway illustrated by Descartes; **Figure 6.3**) was this: damage occurs to a part of your body, pain signals go to the brain, you feel pain, you respond by moving away from harm. This is the outdated theory.

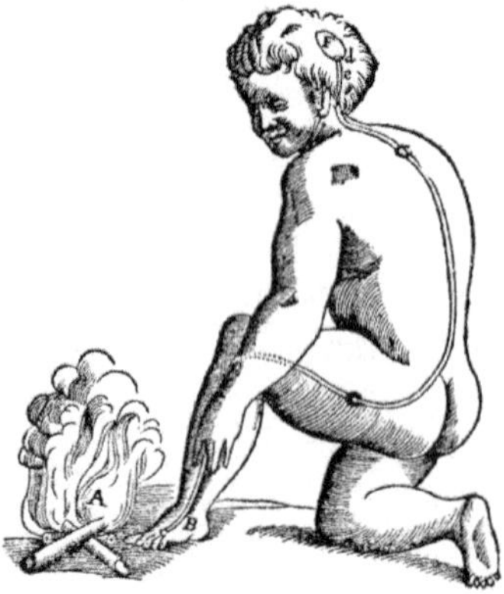

Figure 6.3: Illustration of the pain pathway in René Descartes' *Traité de l'homme* (Treatise of Man), 1664. *Source*: Wellcome Library. Public domain via Wikimedia Commons.

The updated version is as follows: damage or potential damage occurs, signals (not pain signals) but just signals travel along nerves through your spinal cord to your brain where they are interpreted. To keep this explanation simple, your brain may interpret them as harmful or not. Your brain decides if pain is an appropriate reaction. Pain is an output of the brain but it is nearly always in response to an input. The brain can also reduce the incoming signals by triggering your brain's own natural pain relief.

By now, hopefully, you can appreciate that pain is not simple and its complexity is due to the brain's involvement. You cannot have pain without the brain.

Positively, this means that it is possible to use our brain to reduce our pain, but because the brain is not under full conscious control, we cannot simply wish pain away and there may still be a physical trigger for the pain. We need to realise and recognise how the brain can alter our experience of pain. Let us step back from the detail for a second while I share a famous pain story with you.

This is a well-known story of a young builder who jumped onto a 18-cm nail that penetrated right through the front of his boot. As you can imagine, this was excruciatingly painful for him and he required strong sedation for the nail to be removed.

After removal of the nail and on inspecting his foot, he realised the nail had gone in-between his toes and his foot was absolutely fine. Thus, in this rare example, the input to the brain was both visual and the sensation of the nail between the toes was interpreted as highly damaging; therefore, the brain's output was lots of pain.

In my physiotherapy clinic, I commonly witness significant pain reduction if a patient is given credible evidence that there is no damage or no serious issues, much like the young builder after seeing his undamaged foot.

Thus, when a signal arrives at the brain that may indicate damage or potential harm, what factors can either amplify or reduce pain output? The answer is potentially everything, including knowledge, sleep quality, your job, social interactions, culture and physical activity levels. Scientists often group these into the following three categories:

- biological;
- psychological; and
- social.

The common collective medical term for these are biopsychosocial factors. Here are some examples.

Biologically, aside from any obvious physical damage, the nerve sensors can malfunction and send incorrect signals to the brain. This would be like a warning light flashing on your car's dashboard but the mechanic cannot find any fault with your engine, instead finding a fault with a sensor. Sometimes a physical problem can trigger a sensor but the sensor then gets more sensitive and 'stuck on' even after the physical problem heals.

Psychologically, depression and anxiety are two of the biggest modulators of the pain experience. Of course, these can also be caused by pain itself; however, recognising them as contributors and seeking professional help is a route to gaining control. It is also widely accepted that stress can affect the body and mind in many ways that increase pain perception. Interestingly, being in love was shown to relieve pain—the study of pain is really very broad!

There are also social factors to consider. Social interactions, what we learn from others, the pain stories they tell us, our culture and the professional advice we receive can also make us feel differently about our pain. So, at this point, I just want to summarise what we have discussed.

Pain is most often triggered by an initial physical problem (but not always—remember the nail!); the relationship between the physical problem and the pain you feel can then start to separate. Our brain can become overprotective, producing pain from harmless stimuli like touch and simple everyday movements.

It seems that the longer the pain persists, the more independent the pain becomes. As the pain becomes more independent, the contribution of the brain increases and the likelihood of a physical trigger is reduced.

In conclusion, even if you are still investigating a potential physical cause of your pain, hopefully now I have made you aware of the other contributors to the complexity of your pain. Hopefully, now you have a better understanding of what pain is and what it is not.

PAIN NEUROSCIENCE EDUCATION

Are your clients interested in learning more about pain?

Pain neuroscientist Lorimar Moseley believes they are, suggesting that individuals can take on 'complex' pain issues, taught via metaphors, examples and images (Moseley, 2003).

However, the majority do not like being told it is all in their mind; although this is neurologically true—pain is an output of the brain—it is akin to saying 'you are imagining it'!

Thus, snappy heuristics like 'pain is an output of the brain' are unhelpful in the clinic; therefore, I recommend using metaphors, analogies and stories to educate patients about pain, such as the builder and the nail.

The use of pain neuroscience education is effective in reducing pain, improving function and lowering fear and catastrophising (Louw et al., 2019). Pain neuroscience education uses stories and metaphors to help individuals rethink their pain experience by understanding the multiple systems and components involved in experiencing pain. The metaphors and analogies help explain the onset and perpetuation of pain and how various factors contribute to the pain experience of the individual.

The metaphors and topics in **Table 6.2** are adapted from the work of Louw et al. (2019).

Table 6.2: Metaphors and topics to educate individuals about pain

METAPHOR	SUGGESTED EDUCATIONAL TOPIC
Your nervous system is like an alarm system to warn you of any danger or potential danger.	Peripheral nerves detection. Impulses are sent to the brain; impulses are interpreted by the brain. Pain does not travel to the brain, only impulses; the brain then decides if the impulses should cause pain.

METAPHOR	SUGGESTED EDUCATIONAL TOPIC
Your pain alarm system can get more sensitive and be triggered by smaller things. This might be like the car alarm triggered by a gust of wind or that time when you could not sleep because of a tiny noise that you had become too focused on.	Peripheral nerve activation threshold reduction. Hypervigilance and brain processing. Nerve pathway strengthening—fire together—wire together. Hyperalgesia.
Seeing is believing. Famous case study of the man who jumped onto a 18-cm nail that penetrated right through the front of his boot and caused him excruciating pain as well as panic in those around him only to find out that the nail had missed his toes entirely.	You cannot see pain on any scan or complex medical devices. Pain is a matter of perception based on sensory input and expectation.
There is no such thing as a perfect body.	Research has repeatedly shown that commonly scanned parts of the body like spines and knees are all different and show signs of relative ageing in people who have reached maturity. Unless there has been recent trauma, it is very difficult to determine if something structural is the cause of the pain experience.
Fortunately, we are not like motor vehicles but that makes us harder to fix. Take any car with any problem to the right person and they will make it work again. This certainty of outcome is just not an option with humans because we are too complex.	Sometimes, we can alleviate pain; sometimes, we can do so only partially but often we need to learn to manage it.

METAPHOR	SUGGESTED EDUCATIONAL TOPIC
The learning alarm. This might be like the car alarm recognising that the motion caused by the wind rocking the vehicle is not changing and altering its sensitivity accordingly.	If a non-damaging stimulus is maintained, the nervous system can habituate to the stimulus and the brain subconsciously; more consciously, you can have a learning experience that shows that a stimulus is not harmful even though it may have initially appeared painful.
Friend or foe?	While it is often unrealistic to suggest patients make friends with their pain, this is an opportunity to suggest than our emotions, beliefs and social interactions all have a proved and significant impact on pain processing. You could explain it as the ability to turn the pain volume up or down.
Hurt may not equal harmed. You can be sore but safe.	It is potentially acceptable to do something even if it causes pain. You can experience pain without danger. Avoiding pain can often make it worse when you do experience pain.
Pain is a normal part of the human experience.	For most people, pain is a normal experience that comes and goes regularly. Some people seem to get through life without experiencing much physical pain at all while others can become troubled by malfunctioning pain systems irrespective of the initial cause.

WHY METAPHORS AND STORIES?

By presenting new information as a story, analogy or metaphor, it depersonalises the communication. The therapist is telling the story and the client listens to it and can choose to relate it to their personal circumstances or not. It is less threatening to their current beliefs than a direct 'let me tell you approach'. Another way of approaching educating the client is to explain that there are three of you: the client, you and the scientists whose information you would like to help the patient make sense of and use to their own personal advantage.

The historical and unfortunately still sometimes current educational approach is more biomedical, featuring anatomical models and structural issues. Think of the classic spine model or image with the crumbling vertebrae and chewy sweet-sized disc bulge. If you have one of these in your clinic, it may be hindering your work and you may wish to discard it. Biomedical pain education is not helpful, has poor efficacy and may increase anxiety, stress and pain through negative expectation and an overall nocebo effect.

In Chapter 5 we discussed the nocebo effect in depth. One important message from the literature is that negative verbal information can convert typically painless stimulations into painful ones and induce nocebo responses as strong as those induced by direct experience (Rodriguez-Raecke et al., 2010). So choose your stories and the words in them wisely.

THOUGHT ANALYSIS (COGNITION APPRAISAL)

We now need to return to the clients' specific thoughts, which are often thoughts that occur rapidly after the onset of pain; they are often termed automatic thoughts or cognitive errors. Notably, clients prefer the 'automatic thought' term. Again, these are not unique to your clients; they are a very human thing. Humans are not rational, we take cognitive shortcuts; believing that you are wholly rational is, in fact, irrational. Some common thoughts relating to pain are shown in **Table 6.3.**

Table 6.3: Cognitions (thoughts) list

COGNITIONS (THOUGHTS)
Pain means that damage is occurring.
This knee pain is because of my running when I was younger.
I will have to stop working.
I need to start looking after myself better.
Arthritis means that the joint is crumbling.

Common thought types

Within automatic thoughts, you can usually identify the following habits. Read the examples and see how many you can recognise in yourself or your clients:

- **Personalisation:** thinking you are individually suffering from an issue affecting a majority. For example, age-associated changes like osteoarthritis being blamed on something you have done rather than the condition's increasing prevalence with general ageing.
- **Magnification:** catastrophising a problem, for example, 'this pain is destroying me' would be a verbal magnification of 'this pain is making me tired'.
- **Selective attention:** pain hypervigilance, for example, the pain is all I can focus on right now.

- **All or nothing thinking:** not returning to activity gradually, for example, a runner who tries to return to running without an adaptive build-up, gets injured, has a set-back and then decides to quit running altogether.
- **Mind reading:** making assumptions of what others think of them, for example, a client suggesting that they are a nuisance and wasting your time.
- **Fortune telling:** making rapid and usually unhelpful future predictions, for example, my hip hurts so it must be arthritis; I need a hip replacement.

The concluding step of the analysis involves inviting the client to assess their personal level of belief in the thoughts identified. To illustrate, consider the thought "pain signifies ongoing damage." On a scale of 0 to 100, where 100 reflects complete conviction, the client is asked to rate their belief. This evaluation is repeated for each thought. It is uncommon for clients to assign a full 100% belief rating to all thoughts, thus leaving a portion of the scale as an indicator of doubt regarding their negative beliefs. This remaining percentage becomes a platform for open discussion, enabling the development of a more constructive alternative belief. The techniques outlined in this chapter can be harnessed to facilitate such discussions.

Evaluation of automatic thoughts

We will now cover how to help clients evaluate their automatic thoughts to determine whether they are accurate. This is often difficult because unhelpful thoughts are often fused with emotion, which increases their belief and probability of defending it against reasonable alternatives. Thus, approach the discussion after a relationship has been established and be sensitive and mindful of your terminology. There is often an element of truth in the statements that should be acknowledged; however, negative emotion all too often distorts thoughts in a maladaptive direction. To help you facilitate this discussion with the client, I next introduce motivational interviewing.

Motivational interviewing (change talk)

Clinical Psychologist William Miller first described motivational interviewing in 1983 (Miller, 1983). He had experienced great success with individuals with alcoholism where other therapists had failed; by reflecting on his methods, he created motivational interviewing. It was advanced further with the help of Stephen Rollnick.

The key assumptions are:

- People have an innate capacity to change themselves.
- One of the biggest influences on client outcomes is the therapist.
- We can predict the influence of the therapist by looking at empathy.

The importance of empathy

Dr Miller noticed that the more a counsellor confronted the client about their behaviour, the more the client drank, indicating that resistance predicts a lack of change. The client should be making the arguments for change, not the clinician, and a healthy relationship is a good predictor of a positive outcome.

The methods and ideas developed from this early work with clients with alcoholism are now widely used in health care.

Resistance predicts lack of change

Using motivational interviewing tactics in practice can be really helpful especially if used early in the intervention. However, we need to move away from being the 'fixer' because our passion to help with advice and suggestions can often trigger resistance from some individuals.

To help avoid this, try to think and explain that 'the client has what they need' and honour their autonomy by prompting them to give you the arguments for change. Key concepts include:

- Partnership—Avoid the expert role.
- Autonomy—Accept and encourage client autonomy.
- Empathy—Have and show compassion for the client as an individual.
- Evocation—Encourage ideas to come from the client.

Motivational interviewing is an effective way of talking with people about change. However, there is no set formula and this would be less effective than being more responsive to the client during a conversation. Despite the variance in how it is delivered, motivational interviewing is evidence-based in a wide range of settings (Rubak et al., 2005). The core skills are represented by OARS:

- open questioning;
- affirmations;
- reflections; and
- summary.

Open questioning encourages the client to express themselves. Examples could include: 'help me understand how your knee affects your life' or 'what needs to change for things to get better'.

Affirmations can be along the lines of 'that is a good strategy', 'you handled the pain really well under the circumstances'. The skill here is for the positive affirmation to be authentic and not scripted. Insincerity will stifle the formation of a good relationship.

Reflections show the patient that you are listening, that you understand; they help to avoid miscommunication. Simply repeating, paraphrasing and seeking confirmation during the conversation can help you achieve this. Examples may include: So you feel that the avoidance of any lifting will protect your spine?; Is it correct that you never engage in any lifting activities?; You always have others lift for you and if that is not an option the item remains in place—is that correct?

Summaries help the client and you form an understanding from your summary of the client's story; within this you need to identify change statements. These are indications that the patient has at least considered change even though they may be ambivalent about it. An example might be: So you have stopped visiting the gym because you feel it may have caused your shoulder pain and that perhaps you should not exercise vigorously at your age? You have been doing gardening and the other day this actually led to your shoulder feeling better for a few days—is that a fair summary?

Can you see a potential change statement emerging here? The client has linked the physical activity of gardening to the reduction in shoulder pain, indicating that they could be persuaded that activity and exercise may help their shoulder further.

If you can incorporate elements of this methodology into your assessments, it may improve your outcomes; just be careful not to try too hard or it can backfire and cause more resistance.

BEHAVIOURAL STRATEGIES

In this next section, we review and reflect on clients' behaviours and actions. Some examples are provided in **Table 6.4.**

Table 6.4: Example of behaviours (actions)

BEHAVIOURS (ACTIONS)
Not putting any weight through a painful joint.
Taking it easy and discouraging my children from running.
Looking for a sitting-based office job.
Looking for a walking group or a gym.
Continuously using a joint even when inactive.

Behaviour and emotions are often improved by initially tackling cognitions.

To initiate behavioural change, first clarify the reported behaviours to reduce misunderstanding and provide opportunity for clients to reflect on them. Help the client identify an alternative behaviour. Ideally, this alternative should come from the client.

Build on successful experiences that have usually already occurred but are buried by the client's generalisation of their pain experience. If a successful experience has not occurred, then you can try to initiate one by setting an achievable short-term activity goal. Another popular option is to combine some manual therapy with exercise to temporally reduce pain and create a single positive exercise experience than can initiate some positive expectation.

EMOTIONS

Next, we consider the clients' feelings and emotions in the context of their presenting problem. Some clients feel comfortable sharing their emotions but others less so; nonetheless, they are important for both types. Examples are provided in **Table 6.5.**

Table 6.5: Examples of emotions (feelings)

EMOTIONS (FEELINGS)
Anxiety about what is really going on inside my body.
Frustrated that I did not know before and worried that my children might do the same.
Sadness over a planned job change.
Positive but anxious about planned changes.
Anxiety and fear of further pain and harm.

Optimistically, emotions should be helped by cognitive and behavioural strategies. A lack of change and emotional resistance may be triggered by a challenge to a core belief. These are much more firmly held integral beliefs that are often expressed as automatic thoughts. The stress associated with ongoing pain can easily trigger a negative core belief. Confronting negative core beliefs can be distressing for clients and the untrained psychologist may make matters worse. This would indicate the need to consider outward referral to a clinical psychologist; in the UK, I may make such a recommendation to the client's doctor.

CONCLUSION

Thoughts, behaviours and feelings really do make a difference to our experience and management of pain. The concepts in this chapter provide the common missing link between the exercise prescriber and their client. While many people will often avoid the psychological elements of assessment because of what can often seem a specialist skill set, this chapter has presented some clear strategies for immediate use. These do not need to be rigidly applied and work best when the information is collected through active listening and general clinical conversation; this way, it is less forced, less contrived and more likely to be authentic.

Dealing with the identified barriers should then pave the way for the start of a successful rehabilitation programme.

REFERENCES

Louw A, Puentedura EJ, Diener I, Zimney KJ, Cox T (2019). Pain neuroscience education: which pain neuroscience education metaphor worked best? *S Afr J Physiother* 75:1329.

Miller WR (1983). Motivational interviewing with problem drinkers. *Behav Cogn Psychother* 11:147–172.

Moseley L (2003). Unravelling the barriers to reconceptualization of the problem in chronic pain: the actual and perceived ability of patients and health professionals to understand the neurophysiology. *J Pain* 4:184–189.

Rodriguez-Raeck R, Doganci B, Breimhorst M, et al. (2010). Insular cortex activity is associated with effects of negative expectation on nociceptive long-term habituation. *J Neurosci* 30:11363–11368.

Rubak S, Sandbaek A, Lauritzen T, Christensen B (2005). Motivational interviewing: a systematic review and meta-analysis. *Br J Gen Pract* 55:305–312.

CHAPTER 7

REHABILITATION CONFLICT

INTRODUCTION

In this chapter, we are going to discuss conflict in the rehabilitation setting and how to avoid and manage it.

I am sure you can think of at least one incident where you had a disagreement with a client, perhaps you misjudged them or they misjudged you or perhaps you just simply felt some tension between the two of you and a lack of common ground.

This can often be due to factors beyond our control. Perhaps the client is from a very different culture to yours or speaks a different primary language leading to regular misinterpretation. The patient may have pre-judged you based on a superficial factor such as age or haircut or other factors over which you have no control.

All we can do is be conscious of the scenarios that commonly cause conflict between clinician and client and proactively seek to lessen the likelihood of these situations arising.

Here are five common things that have the potential to cause conflict between you and your clients.

EXERCISE METHODS

Exercise methods should largely be determined by exercise preferences if the aim is to promote longer-term adherence to a rehabilitation plan. Later in this chapter, we discuss personality matching and introduce the work of Suzannah Brue, who promoted the idea that people have different approaches to exercise and that this is linked to their personality.

One of the fundamental principles is to set exercise methods that suit your client and not your own enthusiasm. For example, you might be a physiotherapist and a keen yoga instructor, but a specific client may not enjoy any yoga-like exercises and prefer more intensive strength training. It may be possible to engage the client in a yoga routine and they may start to enjoy yoga; however, the chances of sticking to the exercise plan would be much higher if the client was given exercise tasks that they are more familiar with and find immediately enjoyable. Therefore, to match the plan to the client, you will need to include them in the decision-making process to choose appropriate exercises. A balance needs to be found between choosing an effective exercise, a preferred exercise and one that is suitably convenient to achieve.

EXERCISE SENSATIONS

This refers to the sensations that the client experiences during an exercise. They may experience pain, clicking, rubbing or grinding. These sensations are disconcerting to them and often lead to cessation of the training session. In terms of pain, the goal is to help them come to an understanding that in the absence of musculoskeletal trauma and in the presence of persistent pain, it is acceptable to exercise while experiencing tolerable pain. In earlier chapters, we covered pain education; in later chapters, we discuss more specifically the outcome of exercise rehabilitation for more specific pathologies even in the presence of pain, clicking or rubbing.

EXERCISE OUTCOMES

Outcome expectations have been described as clinical gold, suggesting that they are a highly valuable piece of information to provide to the client. It is generally well accepted that an optimistic and positive approach from the clinician has an impact on the success of any intervention, providing a placebo effect (discussed in Chapter 5).

As rehabilitators, we need to be aware of outcome mismatches, when a client expects a higher level of recovery than is reasonable. For example, if a client experiences 90% pain relief after 6 weeks of shoulder rehabilitation for shoulder pain, they may report that 'it still hurts' and 'there must still be a structural cause'; perhaps they then request more scans and a surgical opinion in the hope of getting 100% pain relief as quickly as possible. Based on the evidence looking at self-reported pain reduction after musculoskeletal injuries, it is very clear that a significant proportion of clients continue to experience symptoms related to their injury well beyond standard soft-tissue healing times.

Matching outcome expectations in practice requires knowledge and good interpersonal skills. Setting a negative expectation would likely cause a nocebo effect while setting a positive expectation is always preferred as long as it is based on the evidence and it is realistic.

The fact is that even the best evidence-based physical therapist will only have a success rate near to the statistical realities of musculoskeletal research.

Another key message here is that recovery is not all about pain. Pain does not need to be a limiting factor; improved strength through activity will have a big impact on health and well-being and more specifically movement confidence.

For those clients who just say 'ah to hell with all these exercises. I have private health insurance, I am going to get an operation', we have a duty to make them aware of the success rates and expected outcomes from such procedures. This is beyond the scope of this chapter, but I will make two general statements:

- Exercise is often well matched against elective surgery for musculoskeletal issues.
- Many individuals are unaware that surgery does not guarantee pain relief.

MAL-ALIGNED GOALS

Set goals with your clients that are meaningful to them. They should feel that it is their goal and have a sense of ownership in achieving it. We discuss goal-setting in more depth in Chapter 9.

LACK OF TRUST

The client may trust you straightaway because of your professional title or reputation. This makes the interaction in the clinic immediately more productive.

If the client needs to build or be convinced to trust you, then accept that this will take time and essentially cannot be rushed. You could aid the process by highlighting your credibility by discussing research or your past experiences with clients.

PERSONALITY MATCHING

Personality matching may sound a bit like a dating and coupling concept but please stay with me. It is really about coaching and personality profiling to improve patient compliance, exercise adherence and maximise treatment outcomes.

The aim is to achieve the following:

1. Improve your understanding of your own personality in relation to exercise.
2. Understand that your client's approach to exercise may differ from your own.
3. Avoid a mismatch between personalities and exercise approaches.
4. Create rehabilitation plans based on the client's preferences.

The simple and common statement 'treat others the way you would like to be treated' is actually not a very helpful way to go about coaching our patients. How you like to be treated may differ from the client's preferences. We have all had clients report dissatisfaction with other therapists; while we can bolster our own egos with these tales, it is often a case of a personality mismatch or clash of personalities, something that commonly stifles relations between provider and client.

Improving our understanding of personality actually starts with ourselves. Understanding our own relationship with exercise provides the benchmark with which to assess the client's approach.

Here are two different examples of exercise preferences. One client may like to receive specific instructions of what to do and may prefer lots of structure, guidance and reassurance. They may only do the exercise that you set and avoid any other forms of exercise because they have other things they would rather do or need to do.

Another client might just need some general guidance and they are happy to investigate and experiment with their own exercises. They keep active and rarely have a structure to their exercise each day.

Trying to impose your approach to exercise rehabilitation when it differs from the approach most comfortable to the client would probably lead to resistance or poor adherence.

Personality testing is most widely used by corporations for recruitment purposes and is now used in sports coaching and sports psychology. One of the most common personality tests is the Myers–Briggs Type Indicator (MBTI), but there are many others and you will find lots of free testing tools online.

BACKGROUND

Carl Jung (1875–1961) was a Swiss psychiatrist who published work on psychological types in 1921. The work was read and adapted by Katharine Cook Briggs and her daughter, Isabel Briggs Myers, who went on to create the MBTI personality profiling tool. The Myers–Briggs Company continues to follow Myers's guiding principle that understanding personality and difference can change the world for the better.

In 2008, Suzanne Brue, an MBTI master practitioner, published her first book on the influence of personality on exercise titled *The 8 Colors of Fitness*.

TAKING A PERSONALITY TEST

Personality tests can be very detailed and costly. This can make them distracting and awkward to use in the clinic, which is why I would encourage the reader to visit The 8 Colors of Fitness website (https://the8colorsoffitness.com/). It is an easy-to-use, client-friendly tool that does not take up too much time.

Start by assessing yourself so you have an idea of your exercise preferences. When asking your clients to complete the assessment, I recommend you set it as a simple homework task. In my experience, clients enjoy finding out the results and this usually triggers a discussion about exercise preferences and previous adherence problems.

I usually call the test an 'exercise preference test'; clients warm to this idea more frequently than the idea of a physical therapist requesting a personality test!

When you complete The 8 Colors of Fitness questionnaire, you will be assigned a primary colour that represents your fitness personality and suggests the forms of exercise you are most likely to enjoy and adhere to.

Once a client's colour is determined, this opens up a conversation regarding their preferences and allows you to develop a customised plan for them, that is, a plan they are engaged with, will stick with and will lead to results.

CONCLUSION

The strategies discussed in this chapter should help you to avoid or manage conflict.

There is an argument for the potential benefits of conflict because without it we simply allow the client to continue on their current path of misunderstanding and mismanagement. The skill is managing the conflict in such a way that it does not become personal conflict, whereby the client may switch to a different provider and continue their search for a 'magic healer'.

REFERENCE

Brue S (2008). *The 8 Colors of Fitness*. Delray Beach, FL: Oakledge Press.

CHAPTER 8

THE PRINCIPLES OF TRAINING 2.0

INTRODUCTION

If you want to start prescribing exercises for your patients, you need to know the key principles to consider when designing an exercise programme. Personal trainers, sports coaches and strength and conditioning specialists all start by learning the principles of training as a prerequisite to designing effective exercise programmes for performance or rehabilitation.

The aim of this chapter is to consider these principles in the context of exercise for pain relief, which I consider to be characteristically different from exercise for performance enhancement. Most individuals who attend a physical therapy clinic want to eliminate, reduce or learn how to better manage their pain; while exercise is an evidence-based way to achieve pain relief, clients are typically less concerned with objective strength and conditioning outcomes and more focused on pain reduction and general functional improvement. If improved strength and conditioning leads to reduced pain, then this is deemed a suitable outcome by the client; however, we should recognise, as described in Chapter 2, that strength improvement and pain reduction are two independent and only loosely correlated variables. Simply put, getting a client stronger will not guarantee a reduction in pain. It is the premise of this chapter to highlight how the principles of training were not designed for exercise for pain relief; in recognising this we can adapt the use of the principles accordingly.

Before we review each of the principles in more depth, I describe them here briefly.[1]

Overload

This principle stipulates that an exercise stimulus should provide enough stress to the tissues or systems to cause a degree of overload that triggers the body to adapt to the stimulus during a recovery period. For example, tibial bone stress caused by walking would lead to adaptive increases in bone density during recovery.

Specificity

This principle dictates that the stimulus should be specific to the required adaptation. For example, trying to improve hip extensor muscle strength with recreational walking would not be a very specific approach. A more specific example would be a cyclist performing squat exercises to fatigue; while this would lead to adaptive conditioning of lower-limb

---

[1] 2.0 refers to the principles in context, that is, the context of pain relief and health care rather than strengthening and sports performance.

muscular endurance, the squat movement pattern differs from that of pedalling a bicycle and therefore lacks specificity. The most specific exercise for a cyclist would logically be cycling. You cannot get more specific than actually doing the movement you are seeking to improve. This is logical but how many of us teach rehabilitation exercises that differ from the task the client is struggling with?

Progression

With adequate recovery, our tissues and systems can adapt to physical stress. For this reason, the stress input must progress to continue to provide a suitable overload stimulus for adaptation. Progression is usually achieved by increasing the frequency, intensity and duration of the stimulus. It is typical to progress just one of these initially to avoid too much overload.

Variety

The principle of variety ensures that a programme offers different stimuli to help maintain continued adaptation and avoid repetitive tissue stress. It is often also considered a psychological principle that helps maintain exercise adherence and avoids boredom setting in.

Reversibility

The principle of reversibility serves to remind us that the removal of a stimulus will lead to a reversal of adaptive tissue and system changes. The research surrounding reversibility, which is surprisingly sparse, also helps us to understand how much we can reduce an exercise stimulus without losing previously gained fitness.

THE PRINCIPLES IN CONTEXT

How relevant are the principles of training for exercise for pain relief?

Overload

Overload is an important principle for soft tissue, hard tissue and physiological adaptation. In the context of exercise for pain relief, the overload principle can be expanded to include psychological and behavioural components. For example, an individual who is avoiding exercise through fear of pain would be encouraged to undertake some exercise in the presence of tolerable pain and discomfort with the aim of creating a learning experience that concludes with them realising that they can do more than they thought they could while experiencing some pain without a lasting negative impact. This would offer an opportunity to expand their functional capacity by initiating behavioural change with the addition of associated psychological and physical changes.

Because the pain-relieving benefits of exercise are not anchored to improvements in strength or endurance, the principle of physical overload could potentially be ignored when designing an exercise for a pain relief programme. For example, the pain-relieving benefits of exercise can occur before physical overload occurs and exercising non-painful areas of the body has been shown to offer pain relief to the non-exercised painful areas. Here we see a potential cross-education or more systemic mechanism at play, either of which suggests that the principle of overload is too simplistic and limiting for the design of pain-relieving exercise plans.

Specificity

Much has been written about specificity in the strength and conditioning literature as an important component to successfully train athletes for performance progression. The basic concept is that the training must be specific and relatable to the task for which performance enhancement is sought.

Musculoskeletal injury research often highlights specificity as an unimportant factor with many different forms of exercise proving beneficial for reducing the pain associated with common joint problems. These research conclusions can often lead us to think that specificity and the type of exercise does not influence outcome and that the client could do any exercise and still see a benefit. In a clinical setting, it is clear that many independent variables exist that may influence exercise outcome; thus, discrediting the importance of exercise specificity in its entirety is not advisable.

So, does specificity matter?

Yes. Arguably, applying specificity to a programme attempts to make it more efficient at providing a stimulus and response in relation to a task or function. To improve the application of specificity in a pain management programme, I would recommend incorporating psychological and social specificity. For example, if a client would feel more confident in a group exercise session, then the specificity would be to offer a group exercise option.

Another example would be if I was giving a client a hip exercise, I would not necessarily teach them an exercise I knew had the highest gluteus medius electromyography output. Instead, I would consider the client's exercise preferences and seek to understand their lifestyle with the aim of giving them an exercise that was convenient, effective and acceptable. This could be termed client-centred specificity and links with Chapter 7 on personality matching.

Progression

Case study

A client came to see me for help and advice for his persistent back pain. They were very motivated to self-manage and keen to learn new 'back pain exercises'. The session concluded with me demonstrating some simple spinal movements for them to try before our next session. When they returned the second time, they brought with them a large pile of aged paper notes. These were their previous exercise instructions from previous physiotherapists and osteopaths dating back almost 10 years. The client had simply added my exercises to their routine and were trying to complete multiple exercises every day. This story is an example of the need to curtail the progression of exercise rehabilitation when it is impractical and no longer serves the end goal.

For a client with a very low exercise tolerance, it would be logical to guide their physical progression to accomplish physical daily tasks with less effort. This can be achieved with incremental increases of the following exercise parameters: the frequency of their exercise routines, for example, could be increased from once per day to twice per day.

We could instead progress a client by increasing the intensity of their exercise sessions, suggesting that they move from an initial feeling of light-to-moderate fatigue to a more intense feeling of fatigue and perhaps up to muscular failure.

We could advise the client to do a different type of exercise that may offer a newer stimulus and therefore adaptation. It is also an option to increase the duration of an individual exercise or session.

When we are advising clients on exercise with the primary goal of pain relief, we need to look at progression from a more biopsychosocial viewpoint.

Rather than just looking to progress the physical attributes of our client, I propose that we view progression from a psychosocial perspective. Therefore, when the client reaches an acceptable level of fitness, function and exercise tolerance, we can then progress towards joining exercise classes, enjoying recreational activities, active social clubs, help integrate daily activity routines and perhaps discuss the desire for any personal physical challenges that may provide an extrinsic goal and a sense of purpose.

This approach to progression is less physical but is more likely to lead to lasting behavioural change.

Variety

Variety is an important principle of training, offering the potential to avoid boredom by avoiding unnecessary repetitious exercises. Incorporating a variety of exercises may also provide an advantageous range of physical stimuli and offer a distribution of loading forces to avoid repetitive tissue stress injuries. Variance also provides the nervous system with more stimulus, thereby leading to greater adaptation.

Variety can be individualised to suit the client. It can introduce an element of fun or gamification into the rehabilitation; depending on the client's exercise preferences, this can be something that is appealing to them.

Reversibility

Reversibility is a very interesting principle that is often overlooked. It is an accepted fact that immobilisation leads to a rapid loss of muscle size and strength. It is also common knowledge that improving strength takes considerable effort over a prolonged period of time, so in the middle there must be a sweet spot that allows people to maintain their levels of strength and fitness by switching to a maintenance programme that is much less energy-intensive but still allows them to maintain the vast majority of their fitness gains. The available research on this matter does not offer a firm guide as to just what this strength maintenance sweet spot might be. The most important variable is the intensity of the exercise. It is possible to maintain fitness and strength levels with significantly reduced training volume if the intensity is either maintained or has a compensational increase.

What might this look like in practice?

- 1–3 sets of a strengthening exercise to failure.
- Repetition range of 10–15 repetitions.
- 2-minute rest between sets.
- Performed once per week.

COMMON MISUNDERSTANDINGS

1: You cannot improve strength by performing lots of repetitions

Doing many repetitions of an exercise is thought to be a training method for improving muscular endurance; therefore, it is often (incorrectly) assumed that it will not improve maximal strength. For example, if an individual is not engaging in any resistance training then the simple addition of some form of resistance stimulus will bring about strength adaptation. Performing 20 repetitions of an exercise may not be as efficient at producing strength gains as lower repetition ranges but it would still bring about positive strength benefits.

2: Lifting heavy weights will not aid endurance

Low-repetition strength training can make lighter endurance tasks feel easier because they are effectively performed at an increasingly lower repetition maximum. Heavy resistance training does not stimulate the cardiovascular system in a favourably adaptive way and heavy weights are often less tolerated by clients unaccustomed to resistance training.

3: You need to visit the gym, a rehabilitation centre or buy some weights

It is a misconception that the overload training principle requires weight training in the form of machines or free weights. Instead, overload can be achieved by simply providing a stimulus that exceeds that which the client is currently accustomed to. This will vary greatly between clients; for many of them, it can include simple body weight exercises.

4: Working hard is the only way to benefit from exercise

Rehabilitation plans may not need to improve strength. Simply performing an activity, engaging muscles and performing movement tasks without overload or the onset of fatigue can bring about many of the positive benefits of exercise, including inflammatory control and pain relief.

5: Special exercises using specific parameters provide the best improvements

Research indicates that exercise can be performed in various different ways and still have a positive outcome in terms of pain and function. Isometric contractions have been compared to eccentric contractions for tendon pain. Walking has been compared to specific spinal exercises for back pain and small amounts of daily exercise have been compared to more traditional strength and conditioning programmes for neck and shoulder pain. Setting specific rehabilitation protocols is increasingly unjustifiable based on current research.

HOW MANY REPETITIONS AND HOW MANY SETS?

It should be clear by now that repetitions and sets may be irrelevant when designing exercise for pain relief programmes. It is, however, pertinent to share the very basics of the traditional repetition and set ranges for strength and conditioning. It may allow you to design a more physiologically efficient training plan or understand a client's current training adaptation.

Neuromuscular activation

This submaximal training approach serves to activate the associated motor neuron pools through the correct repetitive execution of a movement pattern. The intensity can be low and involve both movement-based and static isometric contractions. The low level of intensity allows neuromuscular exercises to be repeated on a regular basis without the need for extended recovery times. **Table 8.1** shows the recommended training parameters.

Table 8.1: Neuromuscular activation guidelines (isometrics can offer the simplest, least painful starting point)

GUIDELINE	DESCRIPTION
Load	Low at 30% + of 1RM or less
Repetitions	30–60 seconds
Sets	1–5
Rest	60 seconds
Weekly sessions	5–7 days
Speed	Moderate-to-slow or isometric
Fatigue	Low-to-moderate, not to failure

1RM, one repetition maximum.

Muscular endurance

This type of strength is most efficiently trained by performing a high repetition range with a suitably low-to-moderate weight up to a level of fatigue. This type of training is often used by endurance athletes and the military. One advantage of training muscular endurance is that it can often be achieved through the use of body weight exercises or with less equipment than other forms of strength training. Table 8.2 shows the recommended training parameters.

Table 8.2: Muscular endurance training guidelines (time under tension should be a focus, not just repetitions)

GUIDELINE	DESCRIPTION
Load	50–70% + of 1RM
Repetitions	12–15 repetitions
Sets	2–5
Rest	1–2 minutes
Weekly sessions	3–5 days
Speed	Moderate and controlled
Fatigue	Moderate to full fatigue

Strength

The most effective and efficient method of strength training uses very-low-repetition ranges to achieve a high level of muscular fatigue. This is achieved by using a high level of resistance; therefore, specialist equipment and a suitable training environment is often required. In clinical practice, if you are aiming to stimulate an adaptive soft-tissue response, then following these parameters for strength training is the most efficient and effective way of achieving this. **Table 8.3** shows the recommended training parameters.

Table 8.3: Strength training guidelines (manipulating the concentric, isometric and eccentric timings can further enhance the training outcome)

GUIDELINE	DESCRIPTION
Load	70% + of 1RM
Repetitions	5–8 repetitions
Sets	2–4
Rest	1.5–2 minutes
Weekly sessions	2–3 days

Speed	Controlled
Fatigue	Full fatigue

Power

Power refers to rapid force production within a short space of time. Adequate power allows the body to move quickly to both produce movement or absorb force. I have included the training parameters typically used in **Table 8.4.**

Table 8.4: Power training guidelines

GUIDELINE	DESCRIPTION
Load	60%+ of 1RM
Repetitions	3–6 repetitions
Sets	2–6
Rest	3 minutes
Weekly sessions	1–2 days
Speed	Fast
Fatigue	Avoid power loss with low repetitions and rest breaks

CHAPTER 9
MOTIVATION AND ADHERENCE

INTRODUCTION

Motivating people to start a rehabilitation programme often requires implementing different strategies and is likely to use a significant proportion of your interpersonal resources. The results from your motivational efforts are very important if you want to experience successful patient outcomes from well-intentioned and evidence-based exercise interventions.

In this chapter, I review the facts and research that support motivational strategies and tackle the common challenge, that is, sticking to the plan.

In my clinic, I consider myself very fortunate. Most of my clients diligently do their exercises, or so they tell me. Research on the subject of exercise adherence challenges my assumptions; in reality, clients probably tell us what we would like to hear rather than doing what we would like them to do.

A clinic-based study by Medina-Mirapeix and colleagues in 2009 looked at predictive factors for home-based exercise adherence for individuals managing neck and low back pain. They concluded that the average level of adherence was as low as 50% or less. More specifically, they found that adherence to exercise frequency and adherence to exercise duration were influenced by both shared and independent variables. Another key message from the research is that we, as health care or fitness professionals, are a significant influencer of our clients' behaviour. I acknowledge that we come into contact with difficult clients who seem unable to change or follow any kind of health-promoting guidance; in such circumstances, possibly while protecting our own ego, we attribute failure to the client and not ourselves. I openly admit that I have done this, and I predict you might have done so yourself. The likely reality is that we may have been, at the very least, partially responsible for our clients' lack of exercise adherence even if it is reasonable to attribute a degree of responsibility to them. As many coaches attest, success is the product of a collaborative effort between coach and athlete. In our context, this would be reflected in the relationship between clinician and patient. Both success and failure are team efforts.

A list of factors known to influence exercise adherence are shown here:

- the suitability of the exercise programme for the client's pathology;
- the suitability of the exercise programme for the client's lifestyle;
- your qualifications, skills and ability to build trust with the client;

- perceived barriers to exercise (these typically include time and facilities);
- the client's self-belief in the ability to achieve success;
- perceived pain intensity and meaning;
- sociodemographic variables, such as age, number of dependants, income, working conditions, to name but a few;
- previous adherence history;
- intrinsic and extrinsic motivating factors;
- social support;
- specific pathologies; and
- environmental factors, such as the weather and access to suitable resources.

GOAL-SETTING

Goal-setting is one of the best-known motivational strategies; if you have ever endeavoured to find out more about goal-setting, you would have likely read about the 'SMART' acronym, that is, specific, measurable, attainable, realistic, and timed.

SMART

In my opinion this creates an objective and actionable goal. Any such goal could be considered impersonal and I would therefore recommend adding a second acronym 'PIE', that is, *purposeful* to the individual, *impactful* for the individual and *enjoyable* in its process or completion.

PIE gives the patient more reason for undertaking their rehabilitation goal and creates a sense of personal attachment and even passion towards its attainment.

An outline for setting goals is provided in **Table 9.1.** You might like to use it to help your patients set their goals.

Table 9.1: SMART and PIE goals form

S	Specific	
M	Measurable	
A	Attainable	
R	Realistic	
T	Timed	

P	Purposeful	
I	Impactful	
E	Enjoyable	

ADHERENCE BARRIERS

Many people start an exercise plan with good intentions only to find that they struggle to adhere to the initial plan. These barriers to adherence can be categorised into barriers for frequency adherence and barriers for duration adherence.

The frequency of engagement may be reduced by factors including lack of time, lack of money, family commitments and other life goals that do not prioritise dealing with the issue at hand. The client's beliefs also have an important role in determining the frequency of their engagement. If a client believes that the rehabilitation will not work or that 'just resting' will bring about a resolution or that surgery is the only way to deal with the problem, then they are far less likely to complete any form of rehabilitation on a regular basis.

The second measure of adherence focuses on the duration of any given session and the ability to complete a planned session. This is most often limited by physical symptoms, such as pain, clicking joints, clunking tendons, a throbbing muscle and all of those physical oddities that cause concern for the average client. Such concerns are often described as forms of hypervigilance, a symptom of a more general anxiety. For example, many of my clients stopped their exercise or activity session due to clicking knees. A patient with clicking knees who feels it is problematic will often express their concern that they do not want to do damage by repeatedly causing their knees to click. Any such or similar concerns will probably increase the severity of their perceived pain. We looked at ways of managing these perceptions in Chapter 6.

LESS IS MORE

One mistake I made early in my career, or even before I finished my training, was to be too overzealous with exercise prescription, providing clients with too many exercises and then continue to add more exercises as a form of progression. Avoid simply adding future prescriptions to a voluminous personal library of stickmen pictures and handwritten notes.

While some individuals may thrive on the prescription of multiple exercises, research informs us that the more exercises we give, the more we reduce the likelihood of adherence to them (Medina-Mirapeix et al., 2009). It is therefore of value to try to understand what number of exercises will best serve an effective outcome. I found on many occasions that the setting of just one exercise can yield excellent results. The effectiveness of this single exercise approach was demonstrated in a shoulder rehabilitation study by Littlewood and colleagues (2015). We will review this work in more depth in Chapter 14.

TOP TIPS FOR GOOD ADHERENCE

These include beginning with a supervised exercise to build confidence, providing education alongside the exercise, offering further exercise supervision at follow-up appointments and aiming to integrate exercise and activity into daily life.

No matter how you issue your exercises, high-definition photos, videos or sketched stickmen. I find that it is not the quality of the image but the quality of the relationship and communication that allow you to turn a lifeless stickman into a spark for change.

IS PAIN ACCEPTABLE DURING EXERCISE AND ACTIVITY?

This is a complex question to wrestle with. We could rely on the research and simply suggest that the answer might simply be yes, but the question deserves more thought and consideration for each individual client. While much has been written about pain management for commonly persistent musculoskeletal conditions, it should not unbalance the importance of assessing for serious pathology or the warning sign that pain provides after trauma.

This book focuses on pain associated with non-traumatic and non-serious causes. This 'common' pain is associated with many of the joint problems we deal with on a daily basis.

While it is acceptable to exercise in the presence of this type of (non-traumatic and non-serious) pain, we need to ask our client if the pain is acceptable to them, avoiding the temptation to simply tell them that it is acceptable.

It has been suggested that the self-reporting of pain to levels 2 or 3 out of 10 for pain perception is acceptable for rehabilitation exercise purposes when pain is reported as persisting. Adding a numerical value and upper limit like this may implicitly suggest to the client that pain is damaging because, by avoiding those higher pain inputs, we are indirectly indicating that such upper pain levels are harmful, which they may be, but we are also preserving the notion that pain always indicates damage. To counter this problem of pain perception, I recommend a more patient-centred approach that encourages the patient to work at an 'acceptable' level of pain or discomfort during activity. Logically, this acceptability has the potential to be greatly influenced by pain education because this would offer the opportunity for the client to learn why pain during exercise and activity need not indicate a structural problem and unnecessarily limit function. To me this makes more sense than just telling clients that 'it is OK to hurt'. I always got the sense that the client's acquiescent nod was not correlated with their internal beliefs when I was setting exercises back in my earlier career days. It is one of the greatest challenges of communication to have your message interpreted correctly.

But of course, not all pain is acceptable. Pain is there for a reason and that reason may or may not have a structural origin. The practical advice I give is that if the pain does not reduce shortly after the exercise and certainly within a 24-hour period, then this would indicate aggravation and be an unhelpful and unacceptable level of post-exercise discomfort.

For some individuals and certain pathologies, there may be a more delayed response to exercise. This is often experienced by those suffering from tendinopathies; the typical pattern starts with the symptoms initially reducing during activity and then increasing after a period of rest. The time frame for these symptom flare-ups is usually 12–24 hours after the aggravating activity.

The best-known exercise-related pain is delayed-onset muscle soreness (DOMS), which typically occurs from unaccustomed exercise and is most often associated with resistance training, particularly with an eccentric focus. I also find that plyometrics are a common cause of significant DOMS for the unaccustomed. Athletes and non-athletes can usually recall a DOMS experience that has the characteristic feature of a 24–48-hour time frame between the exercise and the often extreme muscle pain and stiffness.

WHAT IF THE PAIN JUST KEEPS FLARING UP?

As we discussed in Chapter 3, some patients may experience an increase in pain after exercise (exercise-induced hyperalgesia). This form of dysfunctional pain regulation provides an additional layer of challenge because exercise does not provide pain relief, it actually increases it, and this is not accepted by the client. Here are a couple of strategies for managing clients who experience hyperalgesia instead of hypoalgesia.

If the client expects or is accepting of a potential post-exercise pain flare-up, this will avoid a mismatch between outcome and expectation. When discussing the placebo effect, I mentioned that a positive outcome expectation was a key ingredient of the placebo effect and yet here I am suggesting the opposite, namely that a negative outcome may occur, to avoid disappointment. There is a clinically significant difference between a realistic and an unrealistic outcome before any positivity or negativity is overlayed on top. For example, how many times have you had clients leave your clinic not fully free from pain and not fully satisfied? In most cases, an immediate full recovery is not possible and to expect this would lead to a disappointing outcome mismatch.

Another strategy is to mention the available research, which suggests that the post-exercise pain flare-up should reduce over several sessions if the client can be encouraged to continue completing the initial sessions in the absence of any early notable pain relief.

A specific research study by Sandal and colleagues (2016) recorded a reduction in exercise-induced pain flare-ups over an 8-week period for individuals undergoing neuromuscular training for hip and knee pain. These results support the theory that accepting some level of pain at the start of an exercise programme will allow the pain-reducing benefits of exercise to occur slowly after multiple exercise sessions.

In my experience, it is getting patients past those first few sessions that is the most challenging.

CONCLUSION

We need to accept that exercise adherence is generally low. For many individuals, exercise adherence should receive more attention than the specifics of the prescribed exercise. This can begin by identifying any barriers the client may experience to starting and maintaining an activity programme. One of these barriers is often pain; although there is a level of acceptability to pain during exercise, this needs to be managed and understood on an individual client basis rather than default pain scale ratings. For some of our clients, they may be struggling to manage and understand exercise-induced pain flare-ups. Using available research and careful guidance, it is possible to reduce pain flare-ups in a sustainable way. Whereas pain medications tend to lose their effectiveness with continued use, exercise seems to increase its effectiveness with continued engagement.

REFERENCES

Medina-Mirapeix F, Escolar-Reina P, Gascón-Cánovas JJ, Montilla-Herrador J, Jimeno-Serrano FJ, Collins SM (2009). Predictive factors of adherence to frequency and duration components in home exercise programs for neck and low back pain: an observational study. *BMC Musculoskelet Disord* 10:155.

Sandal LF, Roos EM, Bøgesvang SJ, Thorlund JB (2016). Pain trajectory and exercise-induced pain flares during 8 weeks of neuromuscular exercise in individuals with knee and hip pain. *Osteoarthritis Cartilage* 24:589–592.

PART 2
REGIONAL REHABILITATION

INTRODUCTION

In Part 1, we covered the science behind why exercise can reduce pain and what to do when it does not. We also introduced theories applicable to the whole body as well as localised dysfunctions. We discussed research relating to the systemic effects of exercise and reviewed the fundamental changes that occur within body systems to facilitate pain relief.

One of the emergent themes was that specificity of exercise selection is not as important when the goals are pain relief and function compared to a sports setting where the goals are performance-based. This has become an overlooked factor during the recent uptake of strength and conditioning knowledge and training by therapists looking to offer their clients extended care beyond passive treatment for pain relief.

While there is evidence to support the notion that specificity in exercise selection is not important for pain relief, it would be poor practice to not consider the specific requirements of the individual and their physical abilities and preferences. I hope I achieved my aim of raising awareness of this in Part 1.

In Part 2 (Chapters 10–15), the aim is to focus on specific regions of the body to provide information on what the best exercises might be for common pathologies. I have attempted to focus on evidence-based exercises that tackle commonly identified dysfunctions. I have tried to avoid showing too many exercise variations or exercises lacking justification. In a clinical setting, after reading the exercise adherence literature, I believe that one effective exercise is much more likely to achieve a successful outcome than a programme of exercises. In cases where clients wish to complete a programme of exercises or participate in a taught class, I still think that specific dysfunctions should be targeted with thoughtful exercise selection that targets either the physical dysfunction or takes into account the client's exercise preferences and lifestyle.

One final important point before we dive into dysfunctions and strategies is the prerequisite to understand and explain to our clients why they are doing the exercise and link this to how to perform the exercise correctly, focusing on the functional aim of each exercise and the learning experience it may offer.

I hope that this and the following chapters provide helpful insights to shape your exercise planning and guide your clients with evidence-informed strategies. You will not find the rehabilitation strategies for all injuries and syndromes but you will learn many strategies that have broad utility across the vast spectrum of client presentations.

CHAPTER 10

EXERCISE FOR ANKLE PAIN

INTRODUCTION

The most common type of ankle injury is an inversion sprain. The mechanism for this is typically the body weight of the individual pushing down over an inverted foot, causing soft-tissue injury and occasionally a fracture. The sprain-to-fracture ratio has been identified as 8:1 (Boyce & Quigley, 2004), so eight soft-tissue injuries to every one fracture from the inversion mechanism.

Inversion sprains account for a large proportion of hospital visits and are the most common musculoskeletal injury. After an ankle sprain, symptoms can persist in about 30% of cases (Van Rijin et al., 2008) and an acute ankle dysfunction can often become a chronic ankle dysfunction, the dysfunction being defined as loss of joint range, pain, reoccurrence of injury and general functional loss. Perhaps unsurprisingly, many individuals do not receive adequate rehabilitation after acute ankle injury (Feger et al., 2017). This chapter will make sure that your clients receive evidence-based rehabilitation after an ankle inversion sprain.

IMMOBILISATION

Before assessment, an injured ankle is often immobilised by pain or the addition of an ankle brace. Immobilisation will continue if a fracture is suspected or confirmed; however, in the absence of a fracture, is immobilisation helpful?

The research reports that outcomes are much better with functional support and exercise compared to immobilisation (Kerkhoffs et al., 2002). A client may present with a self-immobilised ankle due to pain and fear of movement and will therefore need persuasion to begin a rehabilitation plan to reduce the chances of long-term problems and re-injury.

EXERCISE

Performing ankle rehabilitation exercises reduces the risk of recurrent sprains (McKeon & Hertel, 2008), reduces swelling (van Os et al., 2005) and leads to a quicker return to work (van Os et al., 2005). Specific balance exercises also reduce recurrence rates (Hupperets Maarten et al., 2009).

So there is little doubt that ankle inversion injuries recover faster with progressive movement and loading than immobilisation and rest. Many ankle exercises, passive treatments and rehabilitation tools are available. The challenge is to identify what the most important pillars of ankle rehabilitation are so as not to miss anything important when creating a plan.

THE FOUR PILLARS OF ANKLE REHABILITATION

The four pillars are based on an excellent ankle rehabilitation review paper by Donovan & Hertel (2012). Their review categorised chronic ankle inversion dysfunction into four impairment domains for assessment and treatment purposes. The approach has successfully served my clients' ankle rehabilitation needs for many years.

Dorsiflexion

Ankle dorsiflexion range of motion is often severely affected after an inversion injury. It is typical to only have a few degrees of motion in an acutely injured ankle. Dorsiflexion should be monitored during recovery by implementing corrective strategies as tolerated and required. It is worth noting that you need 10 degrees of dorsiflexion for a normal gait pattern when walking and 20–30 degrees of dorsiflexion for running. After successful rehabilitation, it is common for the ankle joint range to remain slightly restricted. However, as long as adequate range has been restored, then function should not be limited.

Assessment

There are a couple of simple ways to measure dorsiflexion, using a standard goniometer or the kneeling dorsiflexion lunge test, sometimes called the knee-to-wall test. **Figure 10.1** shows a visual demonstration with some accompanying instructions below it. I am often asked what a normal toe-to-wall measurement should be. I sometimes suggest a figure of 10 cm based on previous readings; however, in the clinic I see a broad range of results and an average figure is of limited assessment value. Do not forget to compare the test result for both sides. In addition to the distance measurement, make a note of any reported pain and the reported feeling at the end of the available range, typically referred to as the 'end feel'.

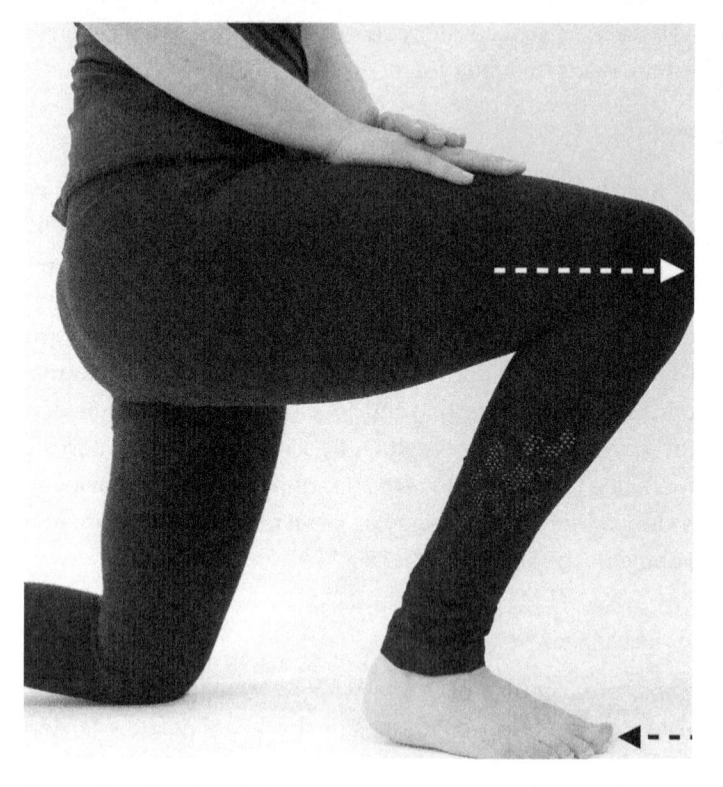

Figure 10.1: The dorsiflexion lunge test is performed by the client actively without footwear. The aim is to document how far the front foot can be placed away from the wall while maintaining the ability to touch the wall with the knee, without the heel lifting. This tests the available dorsiflexion at the ankle and is measured from the tip of the big toe to the wall.

Rehabilitation

There is a simple rule in rehabilitation that if a client fails a physical test, then that test should become the exercise; put more simply, the test becomes the exercise. Therefore, if a client demonstrates dorsiflexion limitation while performing the dorsiflexion lunge test, then this movement can form the foundation of the rehabilitation exercise. Below are two proven rehabilitation techniques for restoring dorsiflexion (**Figures 10.2** and **10.3**).

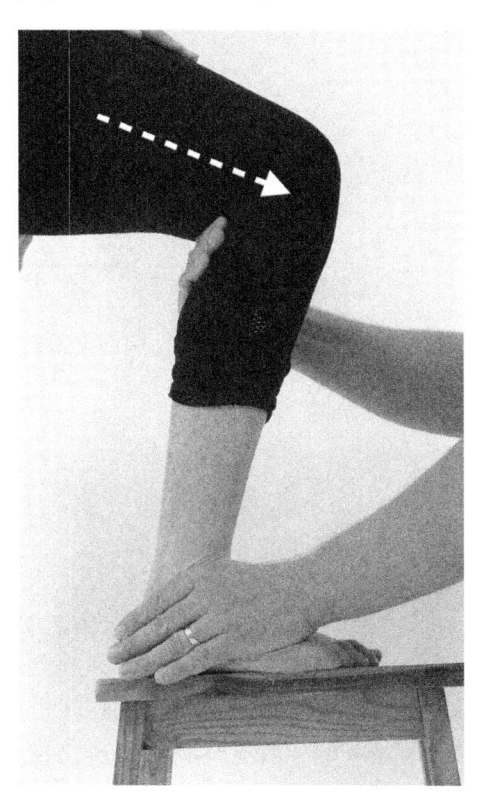

Figure 10.2: With the ankle on a raised surface, it will be easier for the therapist to provide a posterior mobilisation just above the ankle joint by providing a posteriorly directed counter-pressure as the client lunges forward. This achieves a posterior glide during active dorsiflexion and can often lead to increased dorsiflexion range during the procedure.

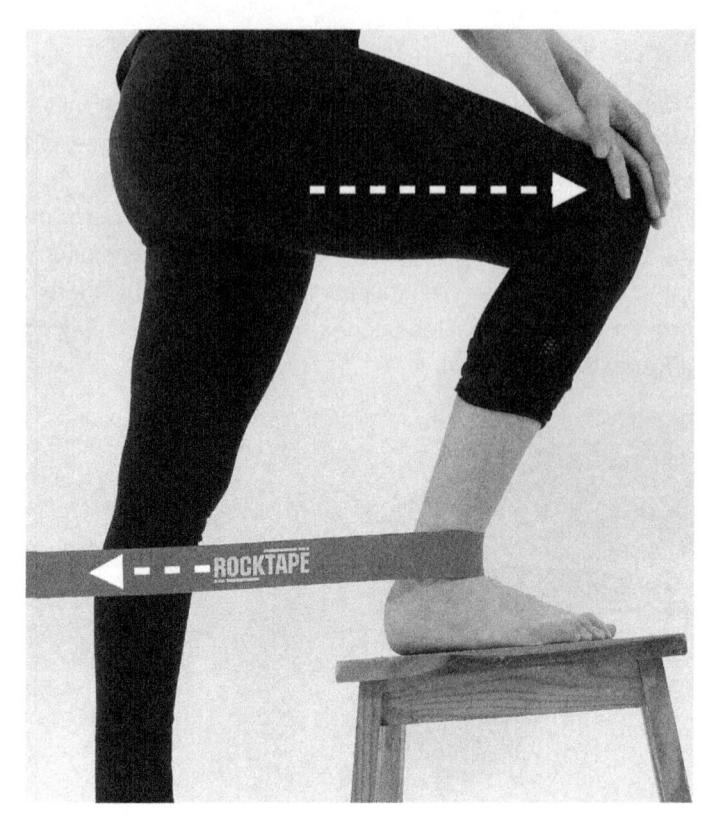

Figure 10.3: Loop a large mobility band over the front of the ankle and ensure it is securely anchored before moving the leading leg forward to create a tension in the band that provides a consistent posterior pull just above the ankle during an active lunge into dorsiflexion.

Top tips from the clinic

Wrapping a rubber therapy compression band around the ankle will improve your grip and is often reported to make mobilisations feel more comfortable for the client (**Figure 10.4**).

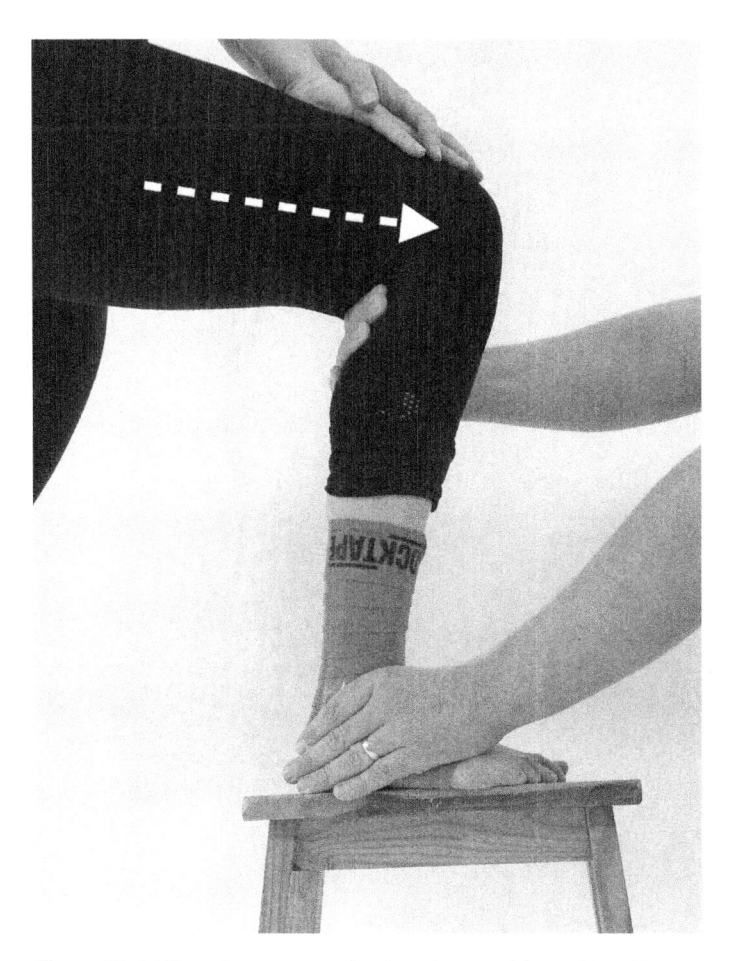

Figure 10.4: Wrap the compression band around the ankle with a low level of compression and a 50% overlap, then tuck the end of the band under the existing band. Because the talocrural joint is mortice-shaped, it will become more structurally stable with increased weight-bearing; therefore, a kneeling lunge position can help to reduce the load through the ankle during a mobilisation procedure. Mobilising into dorsiflexion at different angles can enhance the outcome of the technique (Figure 10.5).

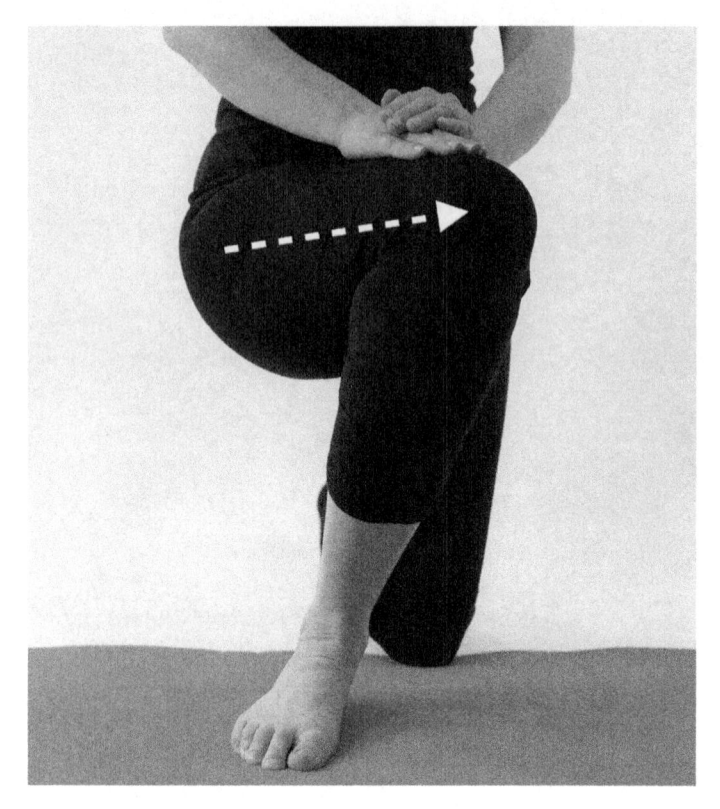

Figure 10.5: Actively mobilise into dorsiflexion at different angles to improve the outcome from the exercise. If a pinching feeling is felt in the anterior ankle, try to adjust the technique by changing the mobilisation angle. Pinching indicates an anterior bony impingement; you should stop any mobilisation that continues to cause these symptoms.

Strength

After a soft-tissue ankle injury, four-way strength deficits have been reported; the normalisation time frame depends on pre-injury strength, with an athlete taking longer to recover adequate strength for return to competition. It is often assumed that eversion should be the focus for ankle strengthening, but with the research reporting a more general strength deficit, it is important to begin a more comprehensive strengthening plan for the ankle that includes resistance training in all directions.

Assessment

Many therapists simply perform some manual testing to provide an opinion on the maximum voluntary force available at the ankle when the foot is pushed against the therapist's hand (Figure 10.6). A more objective and inexpensive test can be achieved by using a simple luggage weighing device (Figure 10.7). More expensive medical tools are available if you require more measurement accuracy.

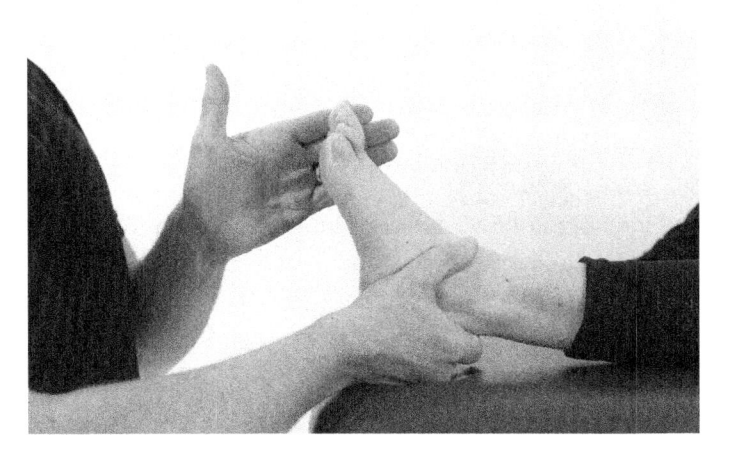

Figure 10.6: A clinical assessment of available strength is often completed with simple manual muscle testing.

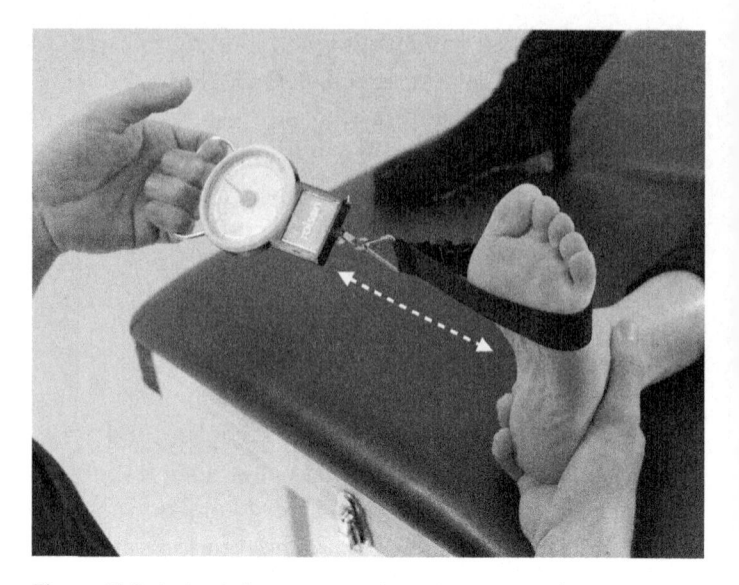

Figure 10.7: A simple luggage weighing device provides an inexpensive strength measuring tool.

Rehabilitation

The simplest way to achieve an adequate resistance into the four movement directions, that is, dorsiflexion, plantar flexion, eversion and inversion, is to provide a fixed resistance in the form of a solid object like a table leg (**Figure 10.8**). Each isometric contraction can be held for 5–15 seconds in each direction. Most therapists prefer to teach dynamic exercises using a resistance band as shown in **Figure 10.9**.

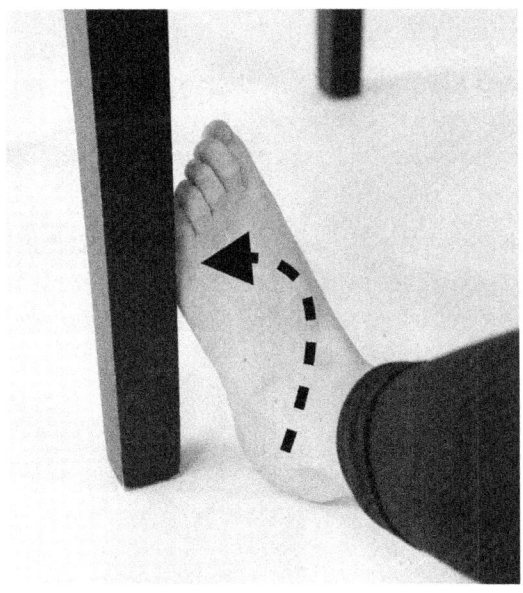

Figure 10.8: Pushing the foot against a table or chair leg can offer a simple isometric exercise to re-engage the muscles around the ankle.

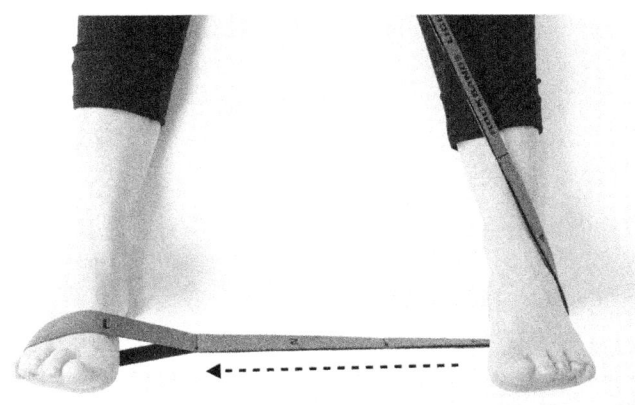

Figure 10.9: A resistance band is being used to provide resistance to eversion ankle motion. The band can then be repositioned to offer resistance in different directions.

Top tips from the clinic

If you choose to teach ankle exercises with a resistance band, make sure you select one with a suitably firm resistance. A flimsy band with little resistance may not offer an adequate stimulus.

To achieve a suitable plantar flexion resistance, teach the client a simple heel raise exercise; pushing against table legs and stretching exercise bands does not usually offer enough resistance to challenge the plantar flexors.

Balance

Initially, balance is reduced bilaterally with the injured side taking longer to restore. This indicates initial alterations in central processing and highlights the importance of balance rehabilitation after an ankle injury. Balance is maintained by three inputs: vision, the vestibular system and proprioception. By effecting any one of these systems you can create a balance challenge for rehabilitation purposes.

Assessment

A variety of recognised balance tests are available; for ankle rehabilitation, I would suggest that you create a simple procedure that consists of 1–3 tests. I typically include the tight rope walk (heel-to-toe walk), standing on one leg and standing on one leg with upper-body weight shifts (Figure 10.10a–c).

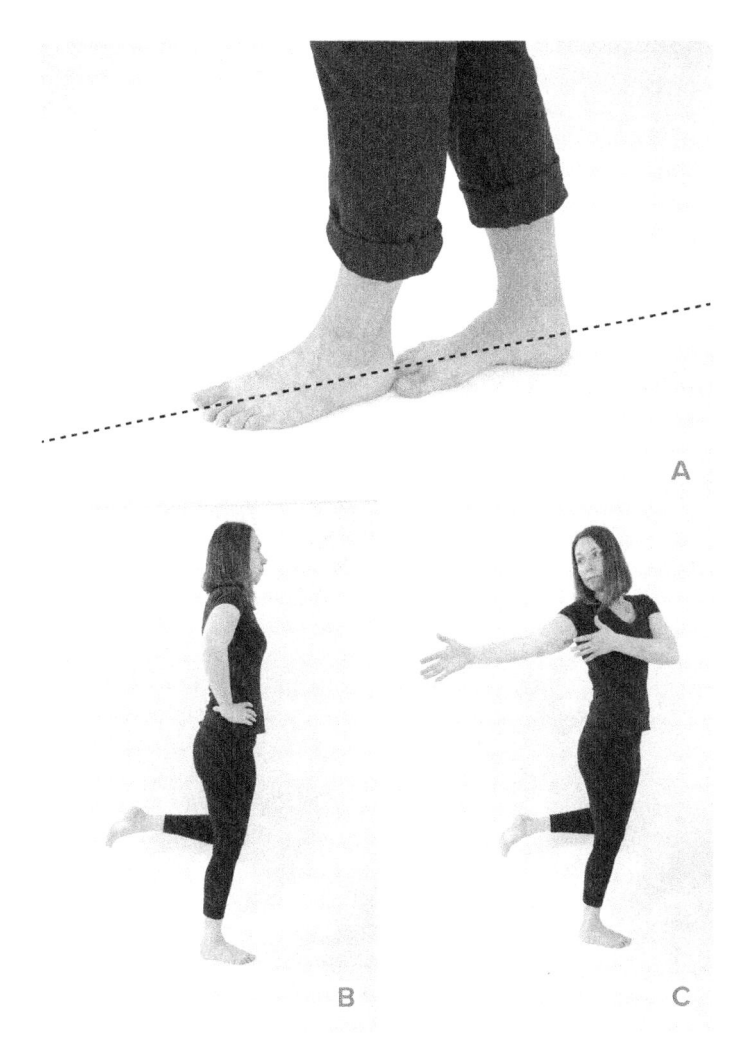

Figure 10.10: Heel-to-toe walk (a), standing on one leg (b) and standing on one leg with upper-body weight shifts (c).

Rehabilitation

These assessment procedures can be used as rehabilitation tasks. Based on the three sensory inputs for balance, further perturbations can be achieved by closing one or both eyes, introducing external motion or by providing extra stimuli like catching a ball or balancing a tennis ball on a racket. A wobble board is a popular option (**Figure 10.11**).

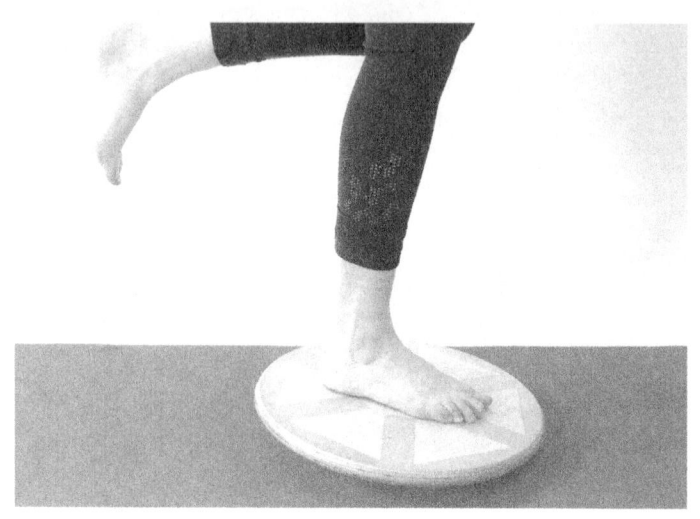

Figure 10.11: An example of a balance task using a wobble board.

Top tip from the clinic

When setting a home balance exercise, try to create one that is interesting and meaningful for your client. I typically get football players to balance on one leg while moving a ball around in a circle with the other foot. For golf players, I create a balance challenge by simulating a swing while standing on one leg.

Gait pattern

After an inversion injury, common functional movements, such as walking, are often altered. Individuals with chronic ankle instability demonstrate altered muscle activation in the lower limb and altered gait patterns. It is important to note that the successful restoration of ankle range of motion, strength and balance may not achieve the return of a normal gait pattern. While the changes during walking may be negligible, such changes are amplified by the increased ground reaction forces that occur during running.

Assessment

The gait cycle can be broken down into stance and swing; these two phases can also be separated into smaller actions, all of which are helpful for assessment purposes. **Figure 10.12** demonstrates the component parts of a normal walking gait cycle, including the different terminology used to describe specific actions.

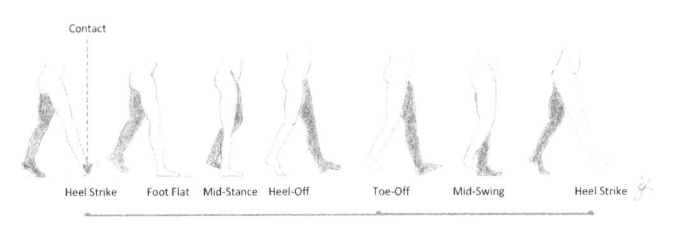

Figure 10.12: The component parts of the gate cycle.

If you are unfamiliar with gait assessment, it can be slightly overwhelming; equally, I have witnessed gait assessment experts that have completely overcomplicated an individual's walking pattern, reporting on all sorts of abnormalities that bear little relevance to the client's problem.

Start by simply deciding if the client is limping; call it an 'antalgic gait pattern' if you must, but perhaps not to the client because the term sounds more serious than 'a limp'. The next thing to do is decide if the limp is caused by a fault in the stance or swing phase. From here, you can specify which component of that phase is deficient. The final task is to determine if the cause is at a localised joint level or the result of a maintained movement habit.

Rehabilitation

The assessment of walking gait should highlight the specific component that needs rehabilitation and whether it is caused by a joint dysfunction or an irregular movement pattern. If a joint dysfunction is detected, this will need to be assessed and managed before reassessing the gait pattern. If movement pattern retraining is required, then this can be achieved by instructing the correct movement using slow repetitions of the component part of the gait cycle. This can then be progressed by repeating the repetitions at a faster speed or by progressing to a full gait pattern that is performed slowly with conscious correction of the specific component part.

Case study

Tony limps due to a shortened stance phase and his pre-swing is shorter due to a lack of toe-off (push-off). Testing reveals reduced plantar flexor strength but no pain and a normal ankle dorsiflexion range. A simple heel raise exercise improves Tony's plantar flexion strength and confidence in his ability to load through the forefoot. Tony is also instructed to perform some toe walking drills and some slow walking with a focus on lifting the heel and pushing through the ball of the feet at the end of each stance phase.

Top tip from the clinic

You can make your gait analysis as complicated or as simple as you like. You can avoid spending any money on assessment equipment or spend many thousands on advanced motion tracking software. However you choose to collect your assessment data, the success of your intervention is contingent on the client being able to implement your corrective strategies, which for most clients requires prioritised, simple and logical instructions.

CONCLUSION

The assessments and strategies described in this chapter are intended to achieve favourable outcomes from ankle inversion injury rehabilitation. They will help to reduce the chances of longer-term problems like stiffness or instability.

The assessments and strategies can also be used or adapted for the treatment and management of ankle dysfunctions caused by different pathologies.

You may have or discover other methods of treating ankle injuries; by making sure you have included the assessment and treatment of the four pillars outlined in this chapter, you can be confident you are providing your client with a high chance of success.

REFERENCES

Boyce SH, Quigley MA (2004). Review of sports injuries presenting to an accident and emergency department. Emerg Med J 21:704–706.

Donovan L, Hertel J (2012). A new paradigm for rehabilitation of patients with chronic ankle instability. *Phys Sportsmed* 40:41–51.

Feger MA, Glaviano NR, Donovan L, et al. (2017). Current trends in the management of lateral ankle sprain in the United States. *Clin J Sport Med* 27:145–152.

Hupperets Maarten MDW, Verhagen EALM, van Mechelen W (2009). Effect of unsupervised home based proprioceptive training on recurrences of ankle sprain: randomised controlled trial. *BMJ* 339:b2684.

Kerkhoffs GMMJ, Rowe BH, Assendelft WJJ, Kelly K, Struijs PAA, van Dijk CN (2002). Immobilisation and functional treatment for acute lateral ankle ligament injuries in adults. *Cochrane Database Syst Rev* (3):CD003762.

McKeon PO, Hertel J (2008). Systematic review of postural control and lateral ankle instability, part II: is balance training clinically effective? *J Athl Train* 43:305–315.

van Os AG, Bierma-Zeinstra SMA, Verhagen AP, et al. (2005). Comparison of conventional treatment and supervised rehabilitation for treatment of acute lateral ankle sprains: a systematic review of the literature. *J Orthop Sports Phys Ther* 35:95–105.

van Rijin RM, van Os AG, Bernsen RMD, et al. (2008). What is the clinical course of acute ankle sprains? A systematic literature review. *Am J Med* 121:324–331.

BIBLIOGRAPHY

Son SJ, Kim H, Seeley MK, Hopkins JT (2019). Altered walking neuromechanics in patients with chronic ankle instability. *J Athl Train* 54:684–697.

DANIEL LAWRENCE

Ankle & Foot Treatment Videos   Ankle Assessment Videos

CHAPTER 11

EXERCISE FOR KNEE PAIN

INTRODUCTION

Knee pain is very common in the general population. In the UK, the prevalence of reported knee pain in adults has been documented at 19% (Webb et al., 2004). Certain pathologies have a higher prevalence in specific subgroups, including sporting, gender and age-defined groups. Osteoarthritis is the most common cause of knee pain in older adults, with degenerative meniscal tears often being included in a degenerative knee diagnosis. Patellofemoral pain is the most common chronic knee problem in younger adults, with an annual prevalence of 23% in the general population and 29% in adolescents (Smith et al., 2018). In this chapter, I also discuss anterior cruciate ligament (ACL) injury, which although clearly a more traumatic injury, is a precursor of post-traumatic osteoarthritis (PTOA). I also offer an answer to a question I commonly get asked on my courses. Is it better to have surgery or not after an ACL reconstruction?

In addition to the prevalence figures, current trends and the recent history of knee pain management represent the typical experiences of clients, which in turn inform client expectations.

I would encourage the reader to avoid the temptation to provide an isolated biomedical assessment and treatment. It is easy to fall into this habit because it remains the foundation of Western medicine for musculoskeletal pain and the search for a physical cause is an accepted norm within Western culture. A great wealth of research is available to inform a biomedical methodology and this is one of the reasons why such an approach is often considered the most credible. While we often hear anecdotally from our clients about their experience of knee pain, this qualitative experience has received significantly less attention in the research; thus, a patient-centred approach often becomes a sideshow to the matinée of a structural diagnosis.

In a pioneering study, Smith and colleagues (2018) reported on the personal experiences of 10 patients with patellofemoral joint pain and identified five themes: (1) impact on self; (2) uncertainty, confusion and sense-making; (3) exercise and activity beliefs; (4) behavioural coping strategies; and (5) expectations for the future. These themes should not be considered specific for patellofemoral joint pain and are relatable to any form of persisting pain. I wanted to use this study as a reminder that although these chapters of the book aim to provide more region-specific exercise advice, it needs to be applied using the knowledge from the previous chapters of the book because even the most evidence-based exercises may be insufficient to address a client's fears and beliefs.

OSTEOARTHRITIS AND KNEE REPLACEMENTS

During the 15-year period between 1991 and 2006, the rate of knee replacements in UK patients more than tripled (Culliford et al., 2010). In the USA, the rate of patients receiving knee replacements demonstrated an even faster increase, with more than an eightfold surge during the 27-year period between 1979 and 2006 (US Department of Health and Human Services, Centers for Disease Control and Prevention, National Center for Health Statistics, 2005).

The cause of this exponential rise in knee replacement surgeries cannot be explained simply by the increased availability of surgery or more efficient procedures (Kim, 2008). It may also be a falsehood to attribute such increases to a higher incidence of knee arthritis. It is conceivable that the uncontested increase in obesity over the last two decades may have contributed to the rise in replacement surgeries, but is such a correlation strong enough to be the primary cause?

Although both ageing and obesity increase the risk of symptomatic knee osteoarthritis, there does not seem to be a matched increase in radiographic osteoarthritis (Nguyen et al., 2011). This suggests that the prevalence of knee osteoarthritis may not have increased in line with the rise in knee replacement surgeries, only the proportion of patients reporting knee pain. This increase in the reporting of knee pain might be caused by an increased awareness of arthritis and the available treatments or possibly an increase in pain reporting in the current generation compared to previous ones. This significant increase in knee joint replacements presents an increasing economic challenge for individuals, organisations and taxpayers. This is a matter of health economic policy and not the aim of this book, so instead I bring to your attention a different but important question.

DO TOTAL KNEE REPLACEMENTS WORK?

The answer to this question often shocks people, regardless of the way it is explained. Many patients have never been openly informed that a knee replacement does not guarantee pain relief.

Imagine you were a patient without any medical knowledge; you can appreciate that this would be a challenging fact to wrestle with. It may be akin to suggesting that putting a new roof on your house might not fix a leak. This seems absurd and would clearly only occur if the new roof was faulty or if the wrong roof was replaced.

As health professionals, we are well aware that a joint replacement may not eliminate the pain because of the poor link between structural changes in the body and perceived pain. We also know that the knee includes multiple components and systems of which the replaced parts constitute only a proportion of what makes a knee function.

Total knee replacement outcome research is highly variable depending on how the data are collected. Data collected by surgeons at their follow-up appointments tend to present more favourable outcomes. Patients often want to show appreciation for the focused attention of the surgeon and their team; they are often given an explanation of their surgical procedure and shown an example or an X-ray of their 'new knee', which often looks better than the 'old knee'. The operation is often described to the patient as a success due to the avoidance of any surgical issues and the successful completion of the operation.

Some patients may be resistant to acknowledge their unresolved knee pain in the hope that it may just be post-operative discomfort. Woolhead et al. (2005) noted in their qualitative study that patients would often report good outcomes from their knee replacement surgery despite also reporting ongoing pain and mobility issues, thus seeming to contradict themselves. While some cases of post-operative pain and dysfunction can be attributed to surgical faults and implant failures, most of the poor pain outcomes are caused by factors that influence pain in general. Factors such as socio-economic status, self-efficacy and levels of anxiety and depression.

The proportion of people with an unfavourable long-term pain outcome after knee joint replacement surgery ranges from 10% to 34%, with a suggested average dissatisfaction rate of 20% (Beswick et al., 2012). With these dissatisfaction figures in mind, it is not simply a case of hoping a knee joint replacement will work. There are identified factors that determine which surgical candidates have a higher risk of unfavourable outcomes. General health status before a joint replacement can influence post-surgical outcome; perhaps less obvious is the influence of the patient's belief system and social support network. We have discussed these patient attributes in Chapter 1 and here we can appreciate that pre-surgical identification and intervention can increase the chances of a successful surgical outcome; the success is then often solely attributed to the surgery.

EXERCISE AND THE DEGENERATIVE KNEE

Osteoarthritis of the knee is best managed using education, exercise and weight control with the addition of medical and surgical interventions when needed (Roos & Juhl, 2012). As shown in **Figure 11.1**, all patients should be offered first-line treatment, while some will need second-line treatment and few will need third-line treatment. Passive treatments include manual therapy, acupuncture and other treatments given by a therapist and not requiring an active lifestyle change by the patient.

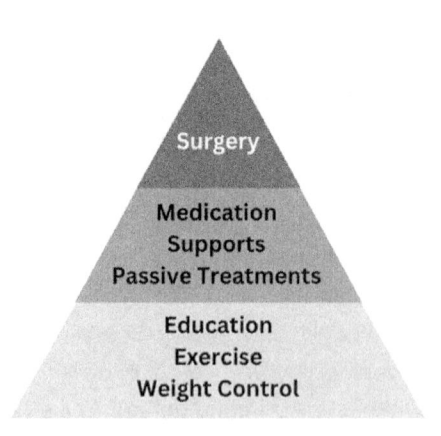

Figure 11.1: The osteoarthritis treatment pyramid. All patients should have the education, exercise and weight control inputs. Some may require additional input in the form of medication, joint supports and passive treatments. A small subgroup may require surgery.

The review by Roos & Juhl (2012) reported that education, exercise and weight loss are effective in the long term and provide a cost-effective first-line treatment. They also noted that all international osteoarthritis guidelines recommend exercise interventions. Furthermore, such programmes show similar benefits regardless of patient characteristics, including radiographic severity and baseline pain.

ARTHROSCOPIC KNEE SURGERY

Knee arthroscopy is also referred to as keyhole surgery, lavage, washout and debridement. It is a common procedure that includes examination within the joint via a small camera, often combined with different surgical procedures that aim to reduce knee pain by washing out or trimming structural anomalies. The procedure can be performed with the general aim of removing excess fluid and loose bodies or with a more specific aim, such as trimming damaged meniscal cartilage. An arthroscopy can be performed purely to examine, without intervention; in some cases, such as some lavage (washout) procedures, it can be performed without an investigative camera; this is not technically an arthroscopy because of the absence of the 'scopy' (meaning viewing, observation or examination).

ARTHROSCOPIC KNEE SURGERY FOR THE DEGENERATIVE KNEE

A degenerative knee diagnosis is often given if joint changes and meniscal degeneration are present. Both occur with or without presenting symptoms at an increasing rate of prevalence in older adults. To some extent, joint degeneration occurs naturally with ageing but it is influenced by many factors, including injury history and lifestyle factors.

Studies comparing knee arthroscopy with sham surgery for the osteoarthritic knee (e.g. Moseley et al., 2002) and for degenerative meniscal tears (e.g. Sihvonen et al., 2013) showed that there is no difference in clinical outcome between a surgical procedure and a sham one.

Research also showed that arthroscopic knee surgery for a degenerative knee, which may include meniscal tears, has no benefit over conservative management approaches in terms of pain, function and the reporting of adverse events related to surgery (Brignardello-Petersen et al., 2017; Lee et al., 2018; Thorlund et al., 2015). When we consider this evidence in clinical practice, it is important to recognise that surgical intervention is occasionally shown to provide a certain degree of patient-reported benefit at the short-term follow-up; however, longer-term follow-up data trend towards matched clinical outcomes at 12 months.

MENISCAL INJURES

Research comparing surgical intervention with sham surgery or comparing surgery to exercise rehabilitation tends to group meniscal degeneration in with osteoarthritis, leading to the common assumption that surgery is not required for meniscal injury. This conclusion is too simplistic and does not provide the clinician with suitable evidence-based guidance. Individual factors such as age, the specific type of meniscal tear and the success or failure of exercise rehabilitation determine the efficacy of a surgical approach. A lack of improvement after 3 months of conservative management indicates the need to reassess the efficacy of surgical intervention.

More severe meniscal damage, such as displaced bucket-handle or flap tears, may require surgery (Bingham, 2020). Advice is best placed, and decisions best made, in light of the available evidence and the wider context of patient expectations.

SURGERY OR EXERCISE?

Clinical practice has responded to the robust research comparing surgery to sham treatment and surgery to conservative management by reducing surgical referrals in favour of conservative management. There is an increasing drive to encourage patients to believe in the efficacy of exercise rehabilitation in place of a previous surgical approach. But how supportive is the evidence base for exercise in the management of degenerative and meniscus-related knee pain, and what outcomes should patients expect?

It is important to recognise that exercise is unlikely to offer 100% pain relief from persistent musculoskeletal problems. This can lead to patient disappointment and the avoidance of exercise if patient expectations are mismatched with the actual outcome.

O'Reilly and colleagues (1999) completed a randomised controlled trial on the effectiveness of home exercise on pain and disability from knee osteoarthritis. The authors reported significantly lower pain scores in the exercise group than in the control group (a reduction of 22.5% versus 6.2%). When we use the 6.2% pain reduction in the non-exercise group as a benchmark, it makes the 22.5% reduction achieved with exercise reflect positively. However, in reality, experiencing only a 22.5% reduction in your knee pain after 6 months of daily exercise may not be heralded as a success by participants. Many patients hold on to belief systems, characterised by uncertainty, about the role of exercise for knee pain, with uncertainty predominantly focused on pain and structural wear and tear (Holden et al., 2012). I believe this is reflected in the common client behaviours we experience in the clinic: poor exercise uptake; not sticking to the plan; repeated visits to the doctor; trying different medications; waiting for scans; focusing on investigative reports; and a perpetual quest for complete pain relief, perhaps occasionally achieved but all too often met with recurrent disappointments and unnecessary health decline.

One of the great challenges we face as clinicians is to guide the client away from unnecessary and potentially deleterious treatment pathways while encouraging positive evidence-informed management approaches that contain realistic outcome expectations. No easy task but one I hope you will find easier after reading this book.

What would you do if you were experiencing the same symptoms as your client? After an injury or when experiencing more persistent symptoms, it is alarming to find ourselves thinking unhelpful narratives of the type we might hear from our clients, while seeking scans and looking for those quick fixes that we spend our days warning our clients about. I do not think this is a sign of being hypocritical; instead, it may reflect how deeply ingrained some of these health beliefs are, perhaps because of our culture and social conditioning.

PATELLOFEMORAL PAIN

Patellofemoral pain is the most common cause of persistent knee pain in younger adults. There are many other knee pathologies that affect adults but what makes patellofemoral pain so unique is the poorly understood aetiology and the stubborn persistence of the symptoms.

In terms of muscle function, sufferers of patellofemoral pain often demonstrate decreased quadricep strength, decreased hip strength and an increased dynamic knee valgus (knock knee), often evidenced by a medial knee drift with single-leg stance during the gait cycle of walking and running. Based on the identified strength deficits, rehabilitation should combine hip and knee strengthening (van der Heijden et al., 2015). Combined hip and knee strengthening provides superior outcomes to isolated knee joint strengthening programmes for patellofemoral pain (Fukuda et al., 2012). If clients are really struggling to load the knee, then isolated hip strengthening can be used to reduce knee pain before introducing knee loading (Dolak et al., 2011). This could be a useful management approach, but you will need to be careful that it does not portray a 'pain equals harm' message to the client by avoiding the loading of the knee.

One of the most disquieting symptoms clients struggle with is the crepitus felt and often heard around the patella. Clients are often dissatisfied with the explanations they receive for the clicking and grinding around the knee, even though there is no link between crepitus and pathology, with crepitus often present in the absence of pathology (Robertson et al., 2010). Many clients experience a cycle of fear avoidance through the inaccurate belief that their crepitus signifies joint degeneration. In addition, clients often report a negative experience of interacting with health professionals regarding their crepitus and feel that it was not taken seriously and was poorly understood as a symptom. To avoid the downward spiral of negative thoughts and reduced movement confidence, it is important that we take the opportunity to recognise the documented failure of health professionals in recognising the significance of our clients' concerns regarding crepitus and clicking joints (not just knees). To date, no link between crepitation and pathology has been demonstrated (Robertson et al., 2017). Clicking usually occurs without pain; however, when an individual experiences pain, they may become more aware of the crepitus and mistakenly associate it to the pain. While there is no clear explanation for joint noise, it is widely accepted that the normal formation and collapse of gas bubbles in the joints' synovial fluid is responsible for the noise. You may find Dr Unger's self-study of interest. The eland antelope is also a unique animal that benefits from its clicking knees (**Figure 11.2**).

For 50 years, a rheumatologist, Dr Donald Unger, cracked the knuckles of his left hand at least twice a day. After 50 years, the knuckles on the left were cracked at least 36,500 times, while those on the right cracked rarely. There was no arthritis in either hand, and no apparent differences between the 2 hands after 50 years.

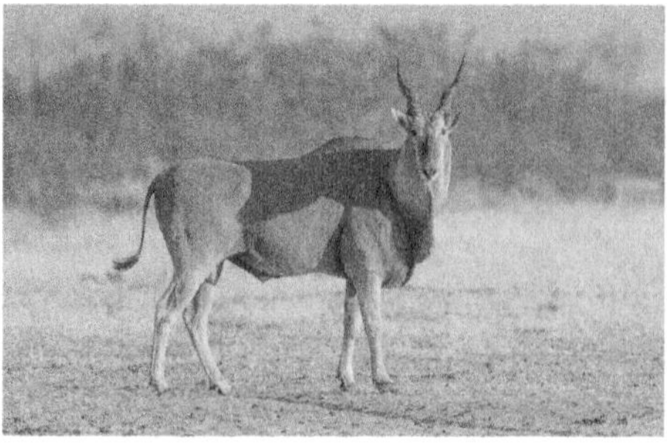

Figure 11.2: The eland antelope uses knee crepitus to display dominance (Bro-Jørgensen & Dabelsteen, 2008). *Source*: Krishnappa YS, Creative Commons BY-SA 4.0 license.

Evidence supports the use of exercise to treat patellofemoral joint pain but does not tell us which specific exercises. While many clinicians believe that patellofemoral joint pain will improve with time, research reports poor outcomes for most individuals after 1 (Collins et al., 2013) and 4 years (Stathopulu & Baildam, 2003).

ACL REPAIRS

After an ACL injury, does a surgical reconstruction lead to better outcomes than a non-surgical rehabilitation plan?

The important outcomes to consider are: post-treatment knee stability; post-traumatic osteoarthritis (PTOA); return-to-sporting participation; pain; and patient satisfaction measures.

Much of the research indicates that surgical reconstruction leads to less reporting of post-treatment knee instability (Rodriguez, 2021). Knee instability also leads to patients opting for surgery many months or years after initially opting for a non-surgical approach. For example, Monk et al. (2016) reported that of the 59 patients in their non-surgical study group, 39% opted for ACL reconstructive surgery at the 2-year follow-up due to knee instability, increasing to 51% at the 5-year follow-up. The authors suggested that there was no difference between surgical and conservative treatment, but this is an unconvincing claim when half of the patients opting for non-surgical treatment opted for surgery at the study's conclusion at the 5-year follow-up.

Another important outcome to consider is whether surgery offers improved protection against the development of PTOA when compared to a non-surgical approach.

After an ACL injury, patients have a high risk of developing PTOA; whether this risk is mitigated with surgery or conservative treatment has been academically debated. As mentioned, surgery appears to offer superior stability outcomes; however, the complexity of the aetiology of PTOA means it is too simplistic to suggest that surgery will lead to less risk of PTOA. Biomechanical research has shown that more motion occurs between the femur and tibia in the medial compartment relative to the lateral compartment of ACL-reconstructed knees (Titchenal et al., 2017), indicating that surgery, as a single intervention, cannot restore normal joint motion. Animal studies also suggested that post-surgical inflammation could increase the risk of PTOA (Heard et al., 2015).

Obesity is a risk factor for many joint pathologies, including PTOA. It is often assumed that the harmful effects of obesity are solely attributed to the increased joint loading caused by excess body weight; however, we now know that adipose tissues release inflammatory substances that have a negative effect on all of our body systems, including joint health.

Obesity is also associated with low activity levels, which limit the weight-bearing stimulus required for cartilage health, predisposing it to thinning. This may create a scenario where obesity has a triple-negative effect on joint health, that is, cartilage thinning, excess loading when active and increased inflammation. There is no debate that weight loss is a proven strategy for reducing knee pain in obese patients. **Figure 11.3** shows the suggested mechanisms of PTOA after ACL injury.

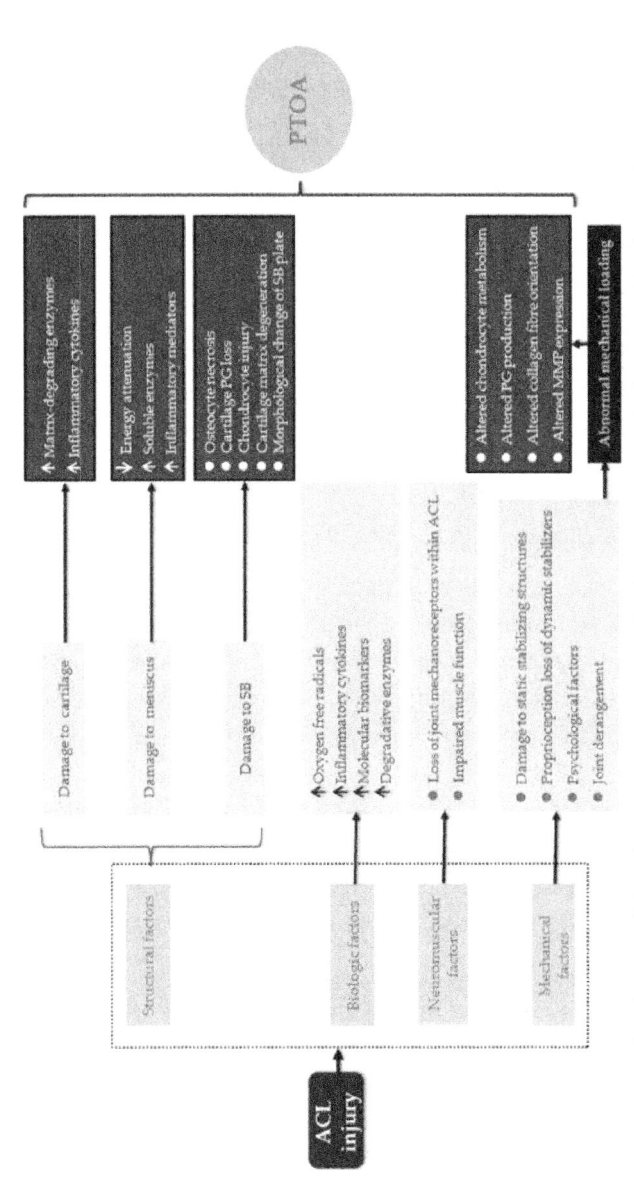

Fig. 1 Suggested mechanisms of PTOA after ACL injury. An up arrow (↑) indicates an increase and a down arrow (↓) indicates a decrease

Figure 11.3: Suggested mechanisms of PTOA after ACL injury. *Source:* Wang et al. (2020). ACL, anterior cruciate ligament; PTOA, post-traumatic osteoarthritis.

After a review of the research, ACL reconstruction remains the preferred treatment approach. This is mostly based on post-injury instability outcomes and not PTOA, which occurs with or without ACL reconstruction. Currently, the best defence against PTOA is prevention of an initial ACL injury (Huang et al., 2020).

DISCUSSION

The effectiveness of surgery to reduce knee pain from various causes is much lower than many patients realise. The two common research findings for elective, and therefore non-traumatic, knee surgery are: surgery often offers no benefit over sham surgery; and a non-surgical approach involving exercise often leads to comparable long-term outcomes.

The efficacy of a surgical approach to knee pain is being increasingly questioned based on the evidence, and the financial cost and health risks involved. However, if health care providers profit from provision, as do all private providers, then this may serve to maintain surgical treatment preferences. Surgery may also be promoted and supported by the organisational structure of hospital health boards, whose care pathways rapidly move patients towards surgical intervention. A culture of surgical intervention is sufficient to maintain higher levels of surgery than the research would otherwise recommend.

After you have trained as a health or fitness professional and gained some experience, it is easy to lose an appreciation for how the patient may view surgery. Surgery is complex, expensive and requires the attention of a highly trained team. The procedure is usually very objective, with a clear plan to physically fix or replace something. In most other facets of life, the best way to deal with a problem is to fix it. It is understandable why patients place such high expectations on knee and other joint surgery, especially if they have been informed that the structure of the joint is the cause of their pain.

Exercise is as effective as surgery for many different types of knee pathology, one of the greatest benefits being the complete avoidance of any of the complications associated with surgery; although only a small risk, it becomes an unnecessary risk when compared to the validity of a non-surgical approach.

The problem that we are faced with, but do not always appreciate from the research, is that the evidence base for exercise rehabilitation is not as convincing as we would like it to be, and not as supportive as many would like. Informing a patient that exercise rehabilitation is as good as surgery sounds very promising, but this is relative to how good that comparative surgery is. There is no doubt that exercise is a very robust tool for managing knee pain but it is not the magic wand we would like it to be. Exercise for knee pain needs to be implemented with a sensitivity for the beliefs and concerns of the patient before the biomechanics and exercise parameters are considered.

Exercise for knee pain

There is an argument for encouraging the patient to do any form of exercise involving the knee, without regard for any specific parameters. However, I provide one evidenced and justified exercise for the knee that I present as the best exercise for knee pain along with justification for doing so.

Slider lunge

The knee joint complex is one of the main weight-bearing joints; it typically functions unilaterally and is aligned by the hip joint's stability and motion. The slider lunge takes these functional factors into account by providing a weight-bearing resistance exercise with a unilateral bias that significantly engages the knee and hip joint musculature. The leading leg provides most of the muscle action; this avoids the weaker limb being sheltered, as can occur with bilateral squat actions or cycling. The front limb should be held in alignment by the hip abductors, which have shown high levels of electromyography activity with lunges and lunge-based exercises. The slider lunge is also a novel exercise for most clients, and one that challenges their balance and coordination and requires more cognitive input than simple actions like squats, cycling or walking. Slide discs are inexpensive but can be substituted for anything that helps the foot slide over the floor.

The slider lunge is an exercise that can be regressed or progressed to suit your clients. It should not be used with a one-size-fits-all approach. **Figure 11.4a–c** shows examples of different versions of the slider lunge to provide options for clients of different abilities.

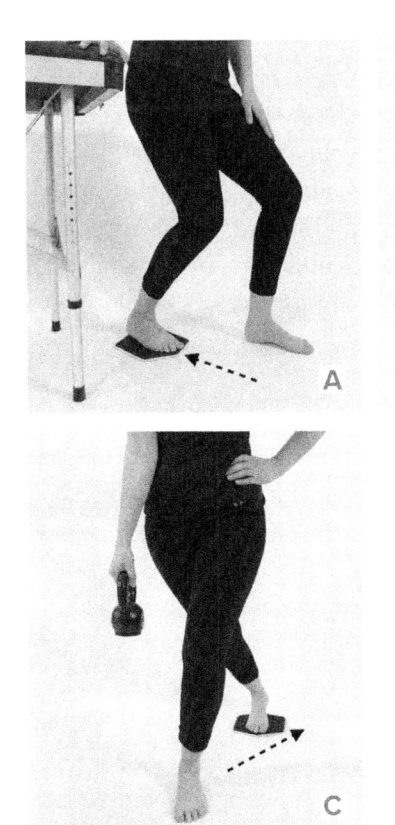

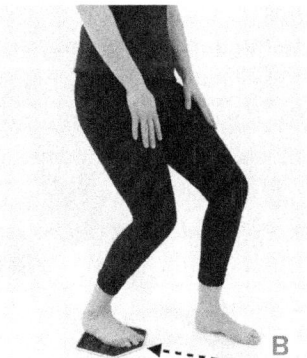

Figure 11.4: (a–c) Three progressive versions of the slider lunge exercise for knee pain. (a) Beginner. (b) Intermediate. (c) Advanced.

Beginner 11.4(a)

Using upper-body support, which is ideal for less physically able clients who may initially lack confidence, make sure that the upper-body support is suitably stable and instruct the client to begin with small lunges initially that focus on flexing the hip rather than kneeling forward. This encourages a more balanced distribution of joint load and muscle strain between the hip and the knee and is often less painful than a knee-dominant lunge.

Intermediate 11.4(b)

Not using upper-body support. This is the standard version of the exercise that most patients should be able to achieve or aspire to fairly quickly. Once the client is able to perform the exercise, it can be progressed by dropping down further into the lunge and slowing down the action to increase the time under tension.

Advanced 11.4(c)

Adding weight or sliding the back leg in different directions (or both). Some clients may require a progressive exercise stimulus, even if only to maintain engagement through the setting of challenges. Adding further resistance in the form of free weights or challenging their balance will create a more advanced exercise option.

REFERENCES

Beswick AD, Wylde V, Gooberman-Hill R, Blom A, Dieppe P (2012). What proportion of patients report long-term pain after total hip or knee replacement for osteoarthritis? A systematic review of prospective studies in unselected patients. *BMJ Open* 2:e000435.

Bingham G (2020). Conservative treatment of meniscus injuries compared to surgical intervention. Poster presentation. *Co-kinetic J* 86:4–7.

Brignardello-Petersen R, Guyatt GH, Buchbinder R, et al. (2017). Knee arthroscopy versus conservative management in patients with degenerative knee disease: a systematic review. *BMJ Open* 7:e016114.

Bro-Jørgensen J, Dabelsteen T (2008). Knee-clicks and visual traits indicate fighting ability in eland antelopes: multiple messages and back-up signals. *BMC Biol* 6:47.

Collins NJ, Bierma-Zeinstra SM, Crossley KM, et al. (2013). Prognostic factors for patellofemoral pain: a multicentre observational analysis. *Br J Sports Med* 47:227–233.

Culliford DJ, Maskell J, Beard DJ, et al. (2010). Temporal trends in hip and knee replacement in the United Kingdom: 1991 to 2006. *J Bone Joint Surg Br* 92:130–135.

Dolak KL, Silkman C, McKeon JM, et al. (2011). Hip strengthening prior to functional exercises reduces pain sooner than quadriceps strengthening in females with patellofemoral pain syndrome: a randomized clinical trial. *J Orthop Sports Phys Ther* 41:560–570.

Fukuda TY, Melo WP, Zaffalon BM, et al. (2012). Hip posterolateral musculature strengthening in sedentary women with patellofemoral pain syndrome: a randomized controlled clinical trial with 1-year follow-up. *J Orthop Sports Phys Ther* 42:823–830.

Heard BJ, Barton KI, Chung M, et al. (2015). Single intra-articular dexamethasone injection immediately post-surgery in a rabbit model mitigates early inflammatory responses and post-traumatic osteoarthritis-like alterations. *J Orthop Res* 33:1826–1834.

Holden MA, Nicholls EE, Young J, Hay EM, Foster NE (2012). Role of exercise for knee pain: what do older adults in the community think? *Arthritis Care Res* 64:1554–1564.

Huang Y-L, Jung J, Mulligan CM, Oh J, Norcross MF (2020). A majority of anterior cruciate ligament injuries can be prevented by injury prevention programs: a systematic review of randomized controlled trials and cluster-randomized controlled trials with meta-analysis. *Am J Sports Med* 48:1505–1515.

Kim S (2008). Changes in surgical loads and economic burden of hip and knee replacements in the US: 1997–2004. *Arthritis Rheum* 59:481–488.

Lee D-Y, Park Y-J, Kim H-J, et al. (2018). Arthroscopic meniscal surgery versus conservative management in patients aged 40 years and older: a meta-analysis. *Arch Orthop Trauma Surg* 138:1731–1739.

Monk AP, Davies LJ, Hopewell S, et al. (2016). Surgical versus conservative interventions for treating anterior cruciate ligament injuries. *Cochrane Database Syst Rev* 4:CD011166.

Moseley JB, O'Malley K, Petersen NJ, *et al.* (2002). A controlled trial of arthroscopic surgery for osteoarthritis of the knee. *N Engl J Med* 347:81–88.

Nguyen U-SDT, Zhang Y, Zhu Y, et al. (2011). Increasing prevalence of knee pain and symptomatic knee osteoarthritis: survey and cohort data. *Ann Intern Med* 155:725–732.

O'Reilly SC, Muir KR, Doherty M (1999). Effectiveness of home exercise on pain and disability from osteoarthritis of the knee: a randomised controlled trial. *Ann Rheum Dis* 58:15–19.

Robertson CJ (2010). Joint crepitus––are we failing our patients? *Physiother Res Int* 15:185–188.

Robertson CJ, Hurley M, Jones F (2017). People's beliefs about the meaning of crepitus in patellofemoral pain and the impact of these beliefs on their behaviour: a qualitative study. *Musculoskelet Sci Pract* 28:59–64.

Rodriguez K (2021). Anterior cruciate ligament injury: surgical versus conservative treatment. *Cureus* 13:e20206.

Roos EM, Juhl CB (2012). Osteoarthritis 2012 year in review: rehabilitation and outcomes. *Osteoarthritis Cartilage* 20:1477–1483.

Sihvonen R, Paavola M, Malmivaara A, et al. (2013). Arthroscopic partial meniscectomy versus sham surgery for a degenerative meniscal tear. *N Engl J Med* 369:2515–2524.

Smith BE, Moffatt F, Hendrick P, et al. (2018). The experience of living with patellofemoral pain—loss, confusion and fear-avoidance: a UK qualitative study. *BMJ Open* 8:e018624.

Smith BE, Selfe J, Thacker D, et al. (2018). Incidence and prevalence of patellofemoral pain: a systematic review and meta-analysis. *PLoS ONE* 13:e0190892.

Stathopulu E, Baildam E (2003). Anterior knee pain: a long‐term follow‐up. *Rheumatology* 42:380–382.

Thorlund JB, Juhl CB, Roos EM, Lohmander LS (2015). Arthroscopic surgery for degenerative knee: systematic review and meta-analysis of benefits and harms. *BMJ* 350:h2747.

Titchenal MR, Chu CR, Erhart-Hledik JC, Andriacchi TP (2017). Early changes in knee centre of rotation during walking after anterior cruciate ligament reconstruction correlate with later changes in patient-reported outcomes. *Am J Sports Med* 45:915–921.

Unger DL (1998). Does knuckle cracking lead to arthritis of the fingers? *Arthritis Rheum* 41:949–950.

US Department of Health and Human Services, Centers for Disease Control and Prevention, National Center for Health Statistics (2005). *National Trends in Injury Hospitalizations, 1979–2001* (No. 2005). Available at https://www.cdc.gov/nchs/injury/injury_chartbook.htm (accessed 19 June 2023).

van der Heijden RA, Lankhorst NE, van Linschoten R, Bierma-Zeinstra SMA, van Middelkoop M (2015). Exercise for treating patellofemoral pain syndrome. *Cochrane Database Syst Rev* 1:CD010387.

Wang L-J, Zeng N, Yan Z-P, Li J-T, Ni G-X (2020). Post-traumatic osteoarthritis following ACL injury. *Arthritis Res Ther* 22:57.

Webb R, Brammah T, Lunt M, et al. (2004) Opportunities for prevention of 'clinically significant' knee pain: results from a population-based cross sectional survey. *J Public Health* 26:277–284.

Woolhead GM, Donovan JL, Dieppe PA (2005). Outcomes of total knee replacement: a qualitative study. *Rheumatology* 44:1032–1037.

BIBLIOGRAPHY

Newsom CT (2017). Surgical vs. conservative interventions for treating ACL injuries. *Am J Nurs* 117:21.

Knee Assessment Videos

Knee Treatment Videos

CHAPTER 12

EXERCISE FOR HIP PAIN

INTRODUCTION

In skeletally mature adults, the hip joint is a robust and congruent joint with significant muscular support and surrounding soft-tissue protection, which is capable of controlling significant loads and has the potential for high levels of mobility. A normal hip joint is rarely the cause of pain in young to middle-aged, moderately active adults.

Hip pain is not common in children and should be carefully assessed, with a low threshold for further investigation. Conditions such as a slipped epiphysis and Legg–Calvé–Perthes disease are rare but serious conditions that would cause progressive and continual hip pain. Childhood hip pain should not be accepted as simple growing pains. Tendon traction pathologies like Osgood–Schlatter disease of the knee and Sever's disease of the heel are common in children and are often labelled as growing pains but there are no equivalent tendon traction pathologies at the hip.

A common cause of hip pain in adults is gluteal tendinopathy or hip bursitis, the latter being a commonly used term but often an incorrect structural diagnosis because the trochanteric bursa is infrequently implicated in lateral hip pain.

Hip pain in younger adults may also be caused by femoroacetabular impingement (FAI). FAI has become an increasingly recognised cause of hip pain that often requires surgical intervention due to the identified anatomical aetiology. We discuss FAI further in this chapter.

In athletic populations, tendinopathies of the upper hamstring tendon, adductor tendons and gluteal tendons provide a common cause of pain that may become chronic if incorrectly managed.

Hip arthritis is the most common cause of reported hip pain in older adults but is three to four times less common than arthritis-related knee pain (Dawson et al., 2004; Linsell et al., 2005). In addition, the reported patient satisfaction levels with hip joint replacement surgery are more favourable than the documented patient satisfaction levels with knee joint replacement surgery. Research reports low levels of dissatisfaction, with figures ranging between 7% and 15% at the 1-year follow-up (Palazzo et al., 2014). Patient dissatisfaction after a total hip replacement is rarely attributable to surgical error and is caused by a range of factors, including outcome expectations, age, sex, secondary health problems, pain management and length of hospital stay (Okafor et al., 2019).

EXERCISE MANAGEMENT FOR HIP OSTEOARTHRITIS

The pain and dysfunction associated with osteoarthritis of the hip can be effectively managed with exercise intervention at all levels of disease severity, including patients awaiting a total hip replacement (Skou & Roos, 2017).

How much improvement in pain and function can a patient expect to gain from exercise? A Cochrane review by Fransen et al. (2014) compared the results of exercise versus no exercise in the management of osteoarthritic hips in a total of 549 participants across 10 selected studies. The systematic review found high-quality evidence that exercise reduced pain and improved function. However, the differences between the exercise and non-exercise groups were described as 'slight'.

On average, the self-reported pain rating was only 8% lower in the exercise group than the non-exercise group. So, although the evidence for exercise was of high quality, it offered only a slight amount of relief. This is important for patients to understand if they are to avoid disappointment. There is also no evidence that exercise modifies the osteoarthritis disease process (Bennell & Hinman, 2011). While there are many credible exercises for the hip joint, I have selected the slider lunge as a starting point and recognise that this was also my recommendation for knee pain. Far from showing a lack of imagination, it is a very conscious exercise recommendation because of the lower-limb positioning and required muscular effort from the hip abductors. The lunge is a functional exercise that loads the hip unilaterally as would occur when walking or running and requires more motor control than a squat action. The lunge action produces one of the highest electromyography readings from the gluteus medius, with the contralateral weighted lunge specifically producing the highest gluteus medius electromyography recording. The addition of the slider disc provides an increased attentional focus and a variable level of skill with many possible progressions or regressions.

THE SLIDER LUNGE

The slider lunge is a lower-limb strengthening exercise that can be adapted to suit different abilities and target different muscle groups (**Figures 12.1**).

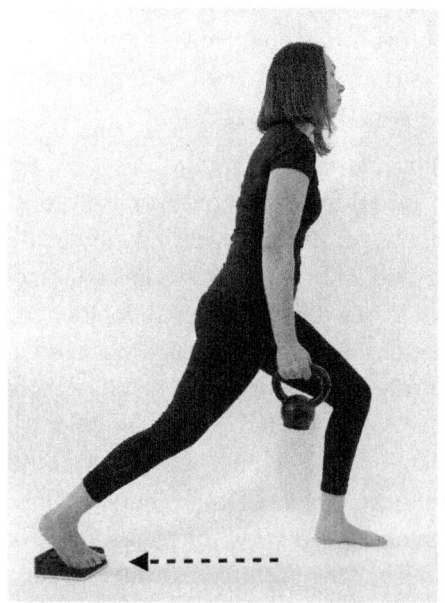

Figure 12.1: Example of the slider lunge exercise showing the addition on an added weight.

SLIDER LUNGE STRATEGIES

The unaffected leg is placed on the slider disc while the affected leg is used to stabilise the body. The disc should then slide backwards slowly and under control while the loaded leg bends at the knee and hip. It is important to control the stabilising leg by preventing hip adduction or internal rotation. If clients experience knee pain, I find this can be reduced by flexing the hips first and sitting back into the movement rather than kneeling forward. While it may be considered acceptable to exercise in the presence of pain, it is by no means desirable. Small modifications to simple exercises can make significant changes to the client's experience of pain.

Upper-body support will allow a regression of this exercise for the less confident or frail individual. In addition, I advise only a partial lowering of the body to perform up to half-range lunges. In most cases, I still encourage the use of a slider disc or similar apparatus because the additional exercise stimulus leads to superior outcomes compared to the more basic lunge.

My preferred ways to advance the exercise include lowering further towards the floor, sliding the disc in different directions or adding a 'destabilising' weight on the contralateral side, as shown in **figure 12.1.**

EXERCISE MANAGEMENT FOR FAI

A multicentre, randomised, controlled trial by Griffin et al. (2018) reported that the treatment of FAI with arthroscopy is comparatively better than a non-surgical approach. Surgery is the favoured intervention for FAI, which is diagnosed in the presence of anterior hip pain, cam or pincer abnormalities on X-ray, and positive provoking clinical tests. The nature of the diagnosis indicates that symptom reduction may be achievable with activity modification and specific exercise selection or avoidance. From my clinical experience, such activity modifications can reduce the likelihood of requiring surgery or help to improve patient comfort while awaiting surgery. The behaviour of anterior hip pain is often such that there is a time delay between aggravating activity and the pain, so that the link between the two is not clear to the patient. Once aware of the suspected joint morphology, patients are much more able to make sense of their symptoms and make changes accordingly.

Table 12.1 shows the best advice to offer clients with FAI and the explanations for that advice.

Table 12.1: Femoroacetabular impingement (FAI) advice

ACTIVITY	EXPLANATION
Avoiding sustained or repeated end-range hip flexion and internal rotation, that is, sitting cross-legged, deep squats, low seats.	These specific positions would approximate a cam or pincer deformity and aggravate the pain associated with impingement.
Resting your body weight on one leg when standing; this is commonly referred to as hanging on the hip.	The weight-bearing leg adducts and internally rotates at the same time as the pelvis drops contralaterally, effectively increasing the adduction and approximation of the femur. Again, this may aggravate the pain associated with impingement.
Side-lying in bed.	If the symptoms of FAI are particularly severe, it is common to experience sleep disturbance due to anterior hip pain of a throbbing nature. This may be alleviated by avoiding side-lying or by reducing adduction with the placement of pillows between the thighs.

ACTIVITY	EXPLANATION
Strengthening the hip abductors.	Weak hip abductors would struggle to control a loaded lower limb and allow more adduction and internal rotation; both motions may aggravate FAI symptoms.
Motor control exercises.	Having an awareness of the positions and exercises to avoid is best taught by learning the exercises that can be performed and how to perform them correctly, for example, teaching a correct squat technique with abduction and suitably limited flexion and a correct lunge without internal rotation of the lower limb.

Factors to consider when squatting are shown in **Figure 12.2a,b.**

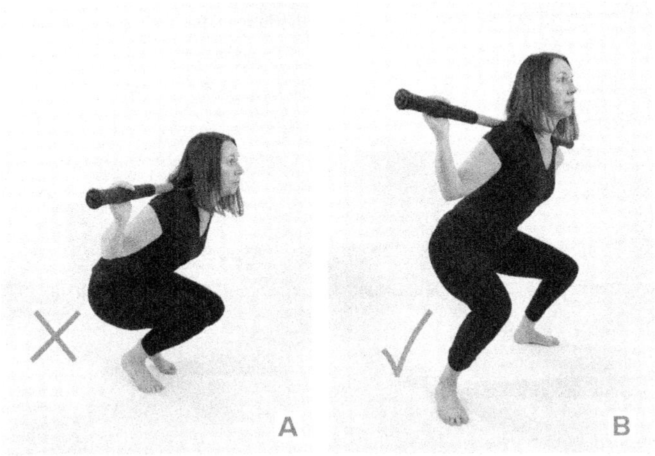

Figure 12.2: (a) Deep squats with the thighs parallel places the hip joint in an internally rotated and flexed position that can cause or aggravate the symptoms associated with FAI. (b) For this reason, clients often find relief from squatting in a more abducted position and not to full depth. In some cases, this simple movement modification can provide the solution.

EXERCISE FOR THE MANAGEMENT OF TENDINOPATHIES IN THE HIP REGION

Exercise and education about load management are proven treatment strategies for tendinopathies; surgery is generally regarded as the last resort for the most stubborn presentations; even then, surgical outcomes for tendon pain are not that promising.

Conservative management, involving exercise, should be considered as the first-line treatment for tendinopathies in the hip region (Frizziero et al., 2016). For gluteal tendinopathy, exercise plus education was shown to be superior to a single cortisone injection or a 'watch and wait' approach (Mellor et al., 2018). Exercise is an important component of hamstring tendinopathy management (Goom et al., 2016), and exercise intervention is evidenced for adductor tendinopathy treatment (Sirico et al., 2020).

EXERCISE OPTIONS FOR TENDINOPATHIES OF THE HIP

Research and clinical testing has led to the selection of the following primary exercises for the three most common hip tendinopathies (**Figures 12.3–12.5**).

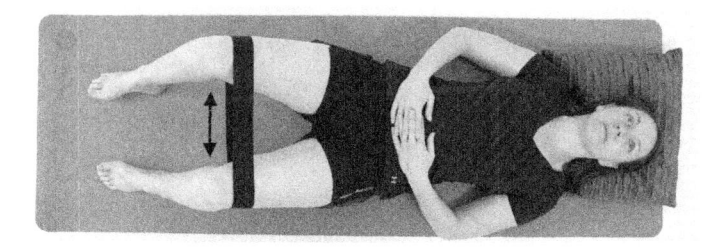

Figure 12.3: The supine isometric hip abduction is a simple exercise to teach for gluteal tendinopathy pain relief; the use of a rigid belt or strap allows clients with different strength levels to complete the exercise. Hip positioning also avoids compression of the gluteus medius tendons over the greater trochanters. The simplicity of the exercise allows the client to perform it correctly. Anything more skilled often leads to less favourable outcomes. This exercise works well if performed for up to 1 minute, 2–3 times per day.

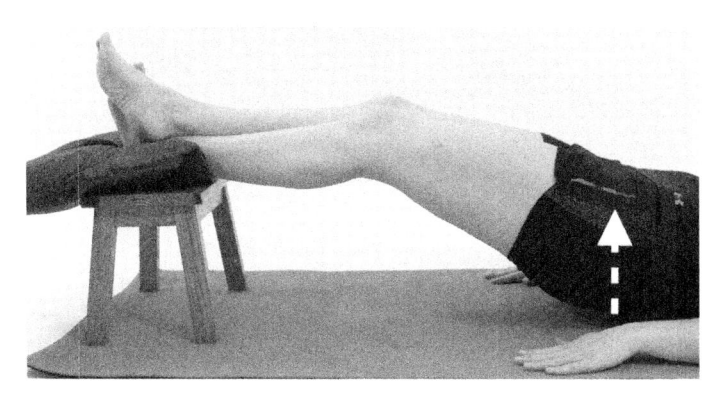

Figure 12.4: The long lever bridge is the favoured hamstring tendinopathy exercise. It allows a controlled loading of the upper hamstring tendons without causing compression over the ischial tuberosities, which can occur with hip flexion exercises. The exercise is best performed with slightly flexed knees while maintaining a neutral spine. Because proximal hamstring tendinopathy is usually characterised by buttock pain when sitting, the use of a pressure cushion when sitting often provides significant relief.

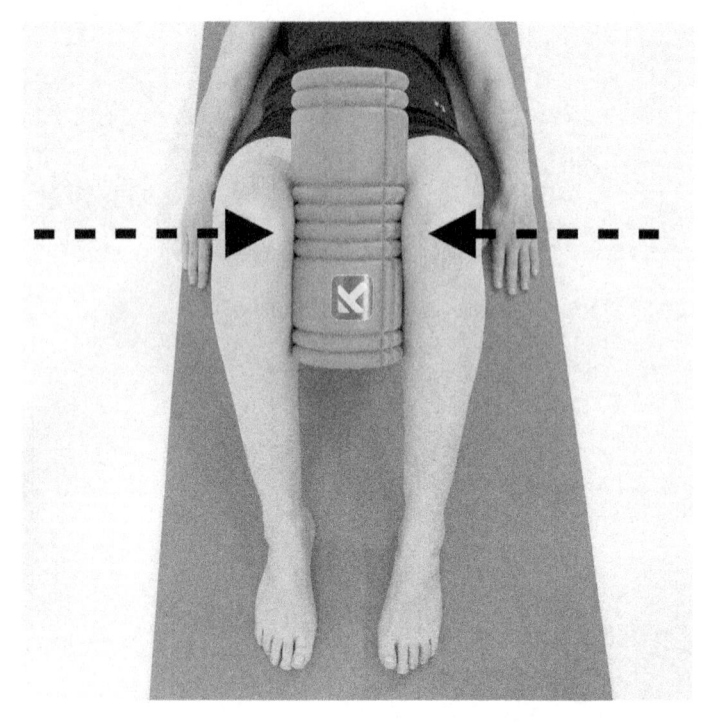

Figure 12.5: Isometric adductor squeezes can be performed for 30 seconds at varying angles of hip flexion and adduction. This simple exercise routine aims to directly load the adductor tendons to initially reduce their sensitivity and initiate a muscle strengthening stimulus.

IMPROVING STRENGTH OR FUNCTION?

It may be helpful for your exercise planning to appreciate that improvements in hip muscle strength may not lead to improvements in movement, especially where the gait pattern is concerned (Willy & Davis, 2011). There is a limited transfer between the different physical attributes measured during rehabilitation. We saw an example of this at the ankle, where improvements in range of motion and strength did not always restore a normal gait pattern. The concept here is that if we identify a movement dysfunction, simply working on the specific muscles or joint responsible for that dysfunction will not guarantee the normalisation of movement. To do this, we need to target the actual movement; in the case of the lower limb, this is usually the gait pattern.

CONCLUSION

For clients experiencing hip pain, I often find it helpful to identify if they are engaging in any repeated or sustained hip internal rotation, adduction or flexion positions that may be causing unnecessary aggravation. Educating the client to avoid these end-range hip positions is likely to reduce hip pain from many of the pathologies presented in this chapter. The simple hip exercises presented in this chapter have been selected from a combination of research and clinical testing; they are not prescriptive or protocols and I encourage you to explore different exercise options. I hope the information and content of this chapter offers relief for your clients experiencing persistent hip pain.

REFERENCES

Bennell KL, Hinman RS (2011). A review of the clinical evidence for exercise in osteoarthritis of the hip and knee. *J Sci Med Sport* 14:4–9.

Dawson J, Linsell L, Zondervan K, et al. (2004). Epidemiology of hip and knee pain and its impact on overall health status in older adults. *Rheumatology* 43:497–504.

Fransen M, McConnell S, Hernandez-Molina G, Reichenbach S (2014). Exercise for osteoarthritis of the hip. *Cochrane Database Syst Rev* 4:CD007912.

Frizziero A, Vittadini F, Pignataro A, et al. (2016). Conservative management of tendinopathies around hip. *Muscles Ligaments Tendons J* 6:281–292.

Goom TS, Malliaras P, Reiman MP, Purdam CR (2016). Proximal hamstring tendinopathy: clinical aspects of assessment and management. *J Orthop Sports Phys Ther* 46:483–493.

Griffin DR, Dickenson EJ, Wall PD, et al. (2018). Hip arthroscopy versus best conservative care for the treatment of femoroacetabular impingement syndrome (UK FASHIoN): a multicentre randomised controlled trial. *Lancet* 391:2225–2235.

Linsell L, Dawson J, Zondervan K, et al. (2005). Population survey comparing older adults with hip versus knee pain in primary care. *Br J Gen Pract* 55:192–198.

Mellor R, Bennell K, Grimaldi A, et al. (2018). Education plus exercise versus corticosteroid injection use versus a wait and see approach on global outcome and pain from gluteal tendinopathy: prospective, single blinded, randomised clinical trial. *BMJ* 361:k1662.

Okafor L, Chen AF (2019). Patient satisfaction and total hip arthroplasty: a review. *Arthroplasty* 1:6.

Palazzo C, Jourdan C, Descamps S, et al. (2014). Determinants of satisfaction 1 year after total hip arthroplasty: the role of expectations fulfilment. *BMC Musculoskelet Disord* 15:53.

Sirico F, Palermi S, Massa B, Corrado B (2020). Tendinopathies of the hip and pelvis in athletes: a narrative review. *J Hum Sport Exerc* 15:S748–S762.

Skou ST, Roos EM (2017). Good Life with osteoArthritis in Denmark (GLA: D™): evidence-based education and supervised neuromuscular exercise delivered by certified physiotherapists nationwide. *BMC Musculoskelet Disord* 18:72.

Willy RW, Davis IS (2011). The effect of a hip-strengthening program on mechanics during running and during a single-leg squat. *J Orthop Sports Phy Ther* 41:625–632.

Hip Assessment Videos

Hip Exercise Videos

Hip Treatment Videos

CHAPTER 13

EXERCISE FOR BACK PAIN

INTRODUCTION

Welcome to the back pain rehabilitation chapter. Here you will find a pragmatic plan to navigate through the myriad of symptoms, systems, randomised controlled trials and clinical protocols in existence today.

This chapter does not provide information on how to assess lower back pain. There are many different methods of assessing the lumbar spine, but the inclusion of spinal cord compression questions (Box 1), also termed cauda equina questions or red flags, should be universal across the professions. Other important assessment questions exist but missed cord compression symptoms can lead to irreversible damage. There is never any harm in revising cord compression signs and they are detailed in **Box 13.1.**

> **Box 13.1: Cauda equina symptoms**
>
> - Saddle anaesthesia: this is characterised by a loss of sensation between the legs (the saddle region), including the genitals and anus.
> - Bladder or bowl disturbance: this involves reduced awareness of the need to urinate, being unable to control urination and loss of anal sphincter control.
>
> Cauda equina syndrome is a rare but serious spinal condition. It needs urgent 'same-day' medical examination and treatment.

THE PAST, PRESENT AND FUTURE

During my career, I have witnessed substantial changes in the management of lower back pain. I have also witnessed absolutely no change! That is to say, while some clinicians dynamically shift their clinical practice based on the latest research and clinical guidelines, others are steadfast in their use of traditional and time-tested techniques.

In reality, most of us sit somewhere along the line that joins these two polarised archetypes. Even the best rehabilitators among us who follow the best guidance and read the best research often fall short of the clinical outcomes we desire. If you need proof of this, you only need to turn to the literature to see that back pain is not a new problem and remains a multifaceted challenge for individuals and society. I am hopeful that the future will bring improved ways to help back pain suffers and I predict that exercise will remain a foundation stone of back pain management, especially as we continue to learn about the complex relationship between exercise and analgesia.

Following the research and guidelines seems a logical path to take, but we have seen national (UK) back pain guidance change many times over the years; much debate exists among back pain researchers, which makes for some confusing reading and less clear guidance overall. Look into the research a little further and it is apparent that a division exists between non-clinical (non-practising) and clinical (practising) researchers. Understandably, clinical researchers have a favourable bias towards the treatment approaches of their professions, which is commonly reflected in research design and conclusions. Non-clinical researchers do not have such a bias and the results of their studies are therefore more valid. You may agree or disagree, but I have heard and read this opinion many times over the years.

An example of our struggle to understand the cause of back pain and the resistance to shifts in knowledge is demonstrated by the stream of research published during the 2000s, which reported that the evidence-based guidelines of the time were simply not working to effectively manage lower back pain. While many studies reported low levels of efficacy for many different back pain treatments, many clinicians argued that research studies often failed to replicate real clinical scenarios by testing just one treatment on a group of patients with back pain presenting with a diverse range of symptoms. The problem could be described as a homogenous approach to a heterogeneous problem or, put more simply, a basic approach to a complex problem. In practice, you would not do the same thing for all of your clients with back pain; if you did, you would deliver that treatment differently depending on the client and their symptoms. The suggested solution to this problem was to subgroup study participants. For example, they may be subgrouped into chronic and acute back pain or flexion and extension dysfunctions or focal back pain and back pain with peripheral nerve involvement. It is also common to subgroup according to range of motion or strength deficits. The problem is that even when you subgroup patients with back pain, the treatments are still rigidly delivered in a way that you would not consider good practice in a clinical setting.

The proposal that lack of subgrouping in lower back pain research accounts for poor treatment outcomes has been challenged by suggesting that the fault may lie with the treatment approach (Wand & O'Connell, 2008) and therefore subgrouping will remain ineffectual.

A second study helps us to continue this narrative by raising awareness that pain and disability outcomes often occur independently of physical performance measures such as range of motion and strength (Steiger et al., 2011). So subgrouping for range of motion or strength deficits is irrelevant if pain reduction is the main clinical goal.

The other ongoing and longstanding clinical debate is whether specific core exercises, commonly associated with Pilates, are better than or equal to general non-specific exercise for lower back pain. The overarching opinion from the research is that 'special' exercises offer no benefit over general exercises (Coulombe et al., 2017; Wang et al., 2012). However, if you analyse the research a little closer, there is a suggestion that specific core exercises may be slightly superior in the short term. There can be many reasons for this. Core exercises are often more physically targeted and mindful. In addition, the very fact that clients often seek a special exercise may play into the hands of a positive outcome expectation for the more prescriptive special exercises. I would advise incorporating both general and specific approaches by combining general daily activities and specific rehabilitation sessions. Even walking has been shown to be as effective as more specific exercise for lower back pain (Vanti et al., 2019). Then again, I think most people know that walking is good for you and that it requires gentle rhythmic spinal motion, so it is not that surprising.

Malfiet et al. (2019) made the following recommendations regarding exercise for back pain:

- All exercise modalities appear effective compared to minimal or no intervention.
- There is no evidence that specific types of exercises are superior to others.
- We should choose exercises in line with the patient's preferences and abilities.
- The effects are better and maintained when combined with a psychological component.

MAKING A START

Let us move forward now and imagine we have a client presenting with lower back pain. We have a wide range of skills, knowledge and research that we can draw on, but how much input do they need?

One popular assessment tool that can be very helpful for determining this is the STarT Back Screening Tool as implemented by Keele University (https://startback.hfac.keele.ac.uk/training/resources/startback-online/).

Complete the nine simple questions with the client, then use the score on the algorithm to determine the risk category. There are specific management interventions for each category and I have summarised these here:

- Low-risk: These clients will often only require a one-off consultation. I usually have a quick in-person or phone follow-up with these clients.
- Medium-risk: These clients often require a short course of physiotherapy or similar.
- High-risk: High-risk clients should receive six individual physiotherapy appointments over 3 months using a combined physical and cognitive behavioural approach.

It is of course important that clients receive effective therapy; being high risk does not mean that the individual needs lots of passive treatment and manual therapy. It means that they need lots of support and guidance and this could include some passive interventions, so long as it primarily supports self-management strategies. There may be many things to consider with higher-risk individuals, such as pain education, functional tasks, exercise advice and occupational management; therefore, these discussions can be rolled out over multiple sessions rather than trying to tackle all components in one session.

THE THREE RS APPROACH

When it comes to rehabilitation, I have had regular clinical success from using the three Rs approach (Norris, 2019). The three Rs refer to the stages of recovery: reactive; recovery; and resilience. The reason I like this approach is because it is based on both the evidence and the clinical expertise of the studies author. In my experience, the concept is also well received by clients, who show a willingness to engage with the rehabilitation plan, especially the resilience phase that is so often ignored.

The three Rs approach suggests many helpful strategies including:

- Use a time goal rather than repetitions or stopping when it hurts.
- Use frequency, intensity, type and time to set and adjust parameters.
- Monitor sudden and post-pain behaviour to manage relapses and avoid catastrophising (behavioural considerations).

GETTING STARTED WITH EXERCISES

After introducing some research on back pain, tools and concepts, it would be easy to remain vague and non-specific regarding back pain and exercise. This chapter shows you some specific exercises to guide you. I am of the firm opinion that it is not the actual exercise that matters, it is why you are doing it, and how you are doing it that can really make a difference to the outcome.

I recommend that you test these exercises on behalf of your clients.

Flow-based routines

Flow-based routines allow you to quickly teach exercise options and progressions. The flow element indicates the aim of fluently moving from one position to another, being mindful but not feeling threatened by the movement. The patient should be cognisant of thoughts and feelings but not controlled by them.

Flexion routine

When we bend forwards, the lumbar erectors relax and lumbar flexion is sustained by passive soft-tissue tension. This is called the flexion relaxation phenomenon (FRP).

The acute onset of back pain often causes a reduced willingness to flex the lumbar spine and therefore causes a loss of FRP due to reported pain and stiffness. The flexion range often returns spontaneously after recovery unless the client develops a fear of flexion and habitually moves in such a way as to avoid it. This loss of flexion can be significantly cemented by poor advice from professionals, friends or something clients have read or overheard. Flexion flow exercises aim to restore the FRP and generally restore available flexion.

Side-lying

We can start from side-lying because this can be the first exercise clients perform in bed when they wake up. Here we can use reciprocal inhibition by contracting the abdominals to flex the lumbar spine; we need to explain that the aim is to curve the lumbar spine and by performing the task slowly and repetitively we can reduce lumbar sensitivity to flexion and progress the range further, or simply reduce the feeling of pain while performing it. The client should aim to complete the movement without showing signs of guarding or threat (**Figure 13.1**). These would be signs like grimacing or breath holding.

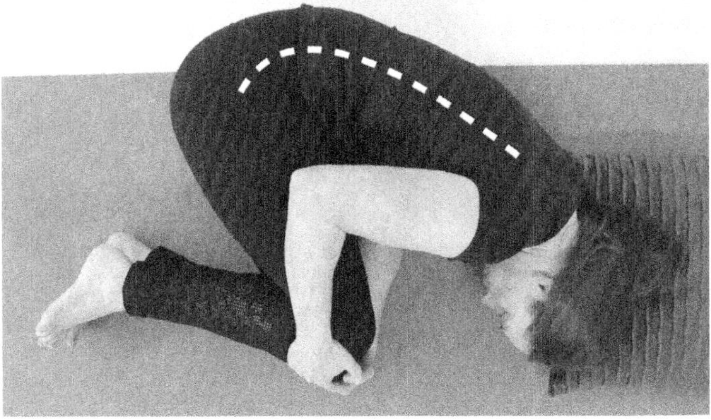

Figure 13.1: Side-lying lumbar flexion exercises can be used to restore lumbar spine flexion without loading the spine.

Supine flexion

No spinal exercise programme would be complete without supine pelvic tilts. This classic Pilates exercise will help to initiate controlled lumbar flexion; I find it is a very useful early intervention for even the most acutely sore lower backs. The exercise starts from a supine position with the feet up (**Figure 13.2a**). The aim is to posteriorly tilt the pelvis, which will flatten the lumbar lordosis, flatten the stomach and increase tension in the glutes. I often describe this as 'flatten the spine,

EXERCISE FOR PAIN RELIEF

tilt the wine'. Just a simple rhyme to help clients remember the action! They need to imagine that a glass of wine is resting on their pelvis and being tilted towards them. You can substitute wine for another beverage, but it may not rhyme.

From this supine position, progress by pulling the knees into the chest and curling forward (**Figure 13.2b**).

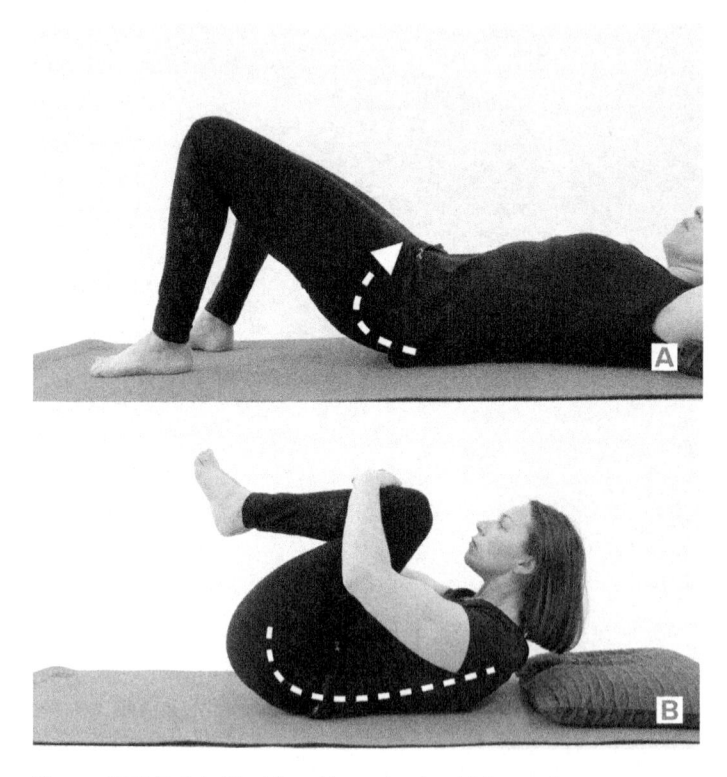

Figure 13.2: Pelvic tilts (a) and knee to chest (b) exercises are popular and typically helpful pain-reducing exercises for individuals suffering with low back pain.

Child's pose

I have had some great results with this exercise in the clinic, which is commonly referred to as child's pose or Balasana in yoga (**Figure 13.3**). I have always found the 'child's pose' title odd; I have children and I have never caught them posing in this position. Despite its odd title, it is a great exercise. You can open the hips into more abduction and external rotation by parting the knees, which will help to clear space for a larger abdomen. You can also exhale to relax into the stretch position and target the lateral sides of the spine by flexing to the sides.

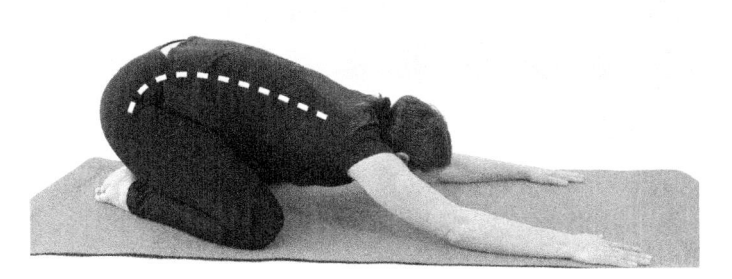

Figure 13.3: The classic Balasana yoga stretch helps to stretch the lumbar spine erector muscles, often alleviating back pain and tension.

Standing flexion roll down

The roll down (**Figure 13.4**) is commonly taught in Pilates classes and is an effective technique for restoring fluent flexion through the spine. The technique can be performed either kneeling or standing. Start with your torso upright in a straight but relaxed position. You should also be relaxed to benefit fully from the exercise. To begin, tuck your pelvis under with a slight posterior pelvic tilt; an abdominal contraction will assist this. The reason we do this is to allow more spinal lumbar flexion from the start of the technique. From this starting position, start flexing the spine from the neck, then let the shoulders come forward and flex through the upper back, progressing to the lower thoracic region and finally the lumbar spine. You can stop here, but I usually progress by allowing flexion through the knees and hips. Return to the upright position and repeat three times.

As a regression, the technique can be performed from a sitting position in a chair. A progression would be the addition of a light weight.

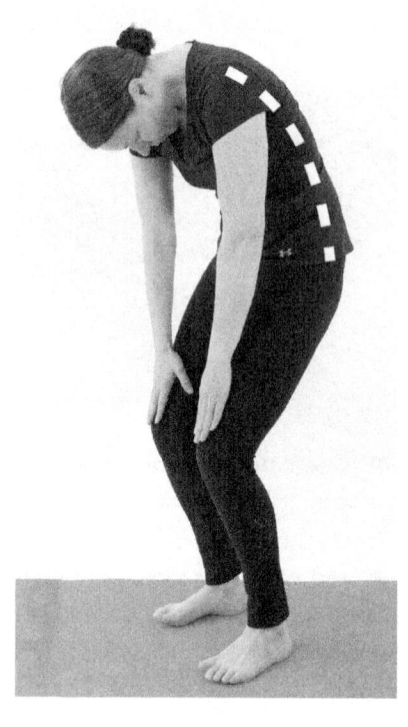

Figure 13.4: The roll down is a dynamic exercise performed standing or kneeling. Breathing control also assists with good execution.

Squat and flex

These next movement flows require more motor control and will need to be adapted to suit each patient. If correctly applied, they can offer the perfect blend of challenge and successful outcome. Be warned that you may fall over the first time you try it! The technique starts in a deep squat then moves between spinal flexion and spinal extension while simultaneously rocking onto the forefoot and lifting up the heels (**Figure 13.5a,b**).

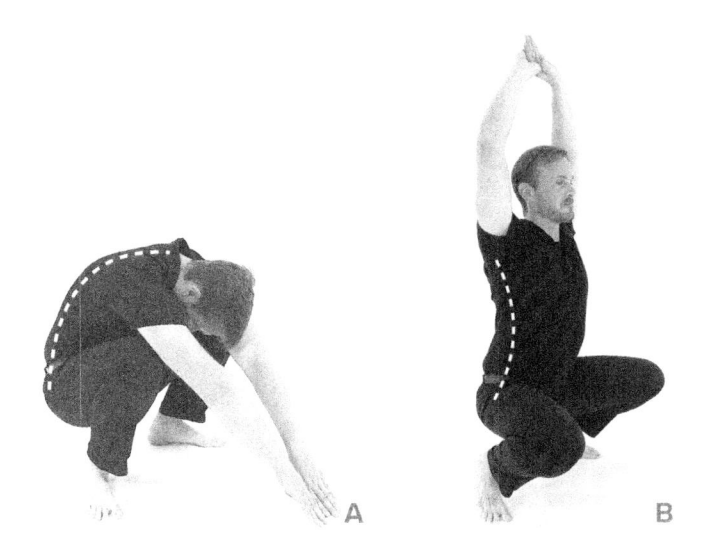

Figure 13.5: The flexion flow routine requires attention to the quality of the motion between lumbar flexion (a) and extension positions (b)

An alternative is to move from a flexion squat up into standing extension. I like to call these the low and high sunrise.

That completes our flexion flow routine. You may have already used some of those exercises in the clinic and hopefully you were introduced to a few new ones.

ROTATION ROUTINE

Rotation range of motion is often measured during spinal assessments and many therapists will rotate the lumbar spine using passive manual therapy techniques. As mentioned previously, walking requires lumbar rotation. The anatomical orientation of the lumbar facet joints leads to joint gapping with rotation. This separation of the joint surfaces can create a cavitation (click or crack) that may have some positive benefits on the nervous system and lead to some transient mobility gains.

Gains in rotation range are also not limited to the transverse plane and it is common for a rotation exercise or treatment to lead to immediate improvements in flexion.

Supine rotation

The easiest way to introduce some rotation through the lumbar spine is the supine short lever twist, often called knee rolling. This technique can be progressed by increasing the leverage with a straight leg and opposite arm extension (**Figure 13.6**).

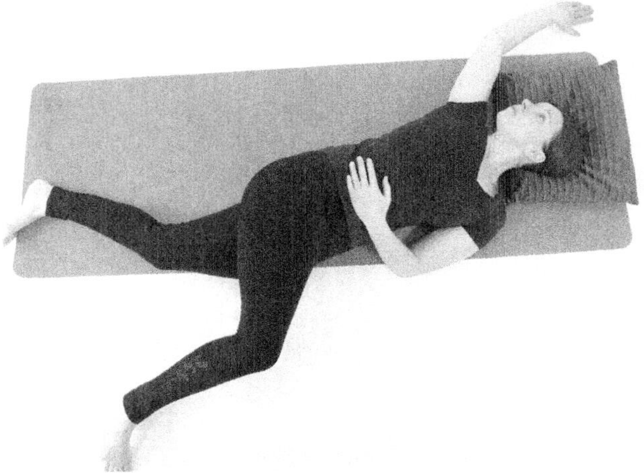

Figure 13.6: Spine rotation using leverage from the arms and legs.

Lunge twist

The lunge twist (**Figure 13.7**) is a simple and effective technique to rotate the lumbar spine. The benefits of this exercise are that you do not need to lie on the floor and you can use your arms over your knee, foot or furniture for leverage to increase the range of motion.

To progress this exercise, you can make it more dynamic by starting in a standing position or repeating it while lunge walking.

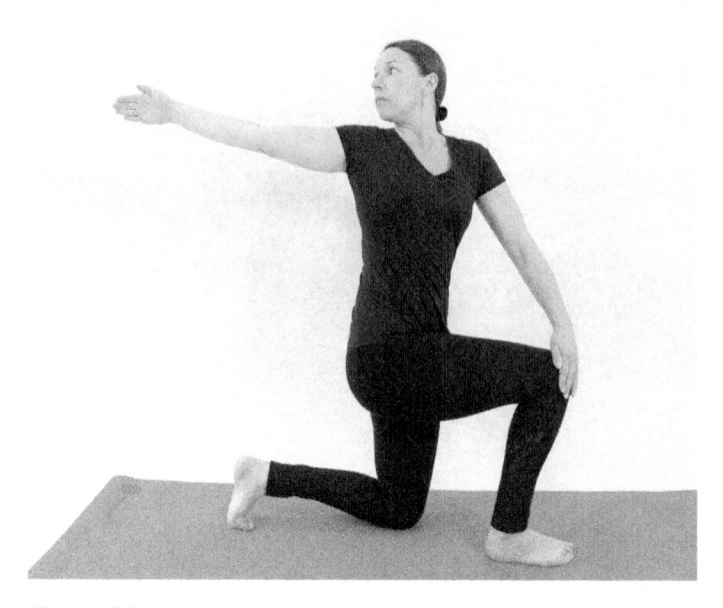

Figure 13.7: The kneeling lunge twist achieves a high degree of rotational leverage if performed correctly.

Walking, with a twist

We discussed how walking has been identified as a beneficial exercise for lower back pain. As mentioned, this may be due to the rhythmic rotational motion it affords the lumbar spine; therefore, we can capitalise on this by accentuating the upper-body rotation when walking, perhaps holding some small weights and completing power walks.

EXTENSION FLOWS

Lumbar spinal extension exercises are not therapeutic for all clients; a patient with acute back pain will often stoop as a pain-avoiding mechanism and forcing extension will only aggravate the symptoms in the early stages. A client with lumbar radiculopathy caused by a posterolateral disc bulge may maintain a flexion with side-flexion to alleviate symptoms. In the older client with lumbar stenosis, patency of the lumbar canal can be improved with flexion to help reduce lower-limb claudication.

So which clients should we extend? Well the general rule is restore what they had before! This may be a little simplistic, but overall, whenever possible, you would want to restore all ranges of motion that the client previously enjoyed. Here are some extension exercises.

Supine hip extension

Lift the hips and relax the abdominals and allow spinal extension to occur, as shown in **Figure 13.8.**

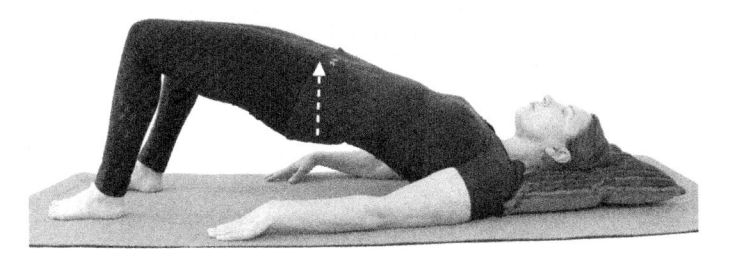

Figure 13.8: The supine back extension exercise.

Prone extension

The 'cobra' stretch is another classic yoga pose called bhujangasana. From a prone position, first extend the spine by resting on the elbows; then, if possible, progress by pressing the upper body up by extending your arms. Lift the head up further and drive the pelvis down into the ground to progress the exercise (**Figure 13.9**).

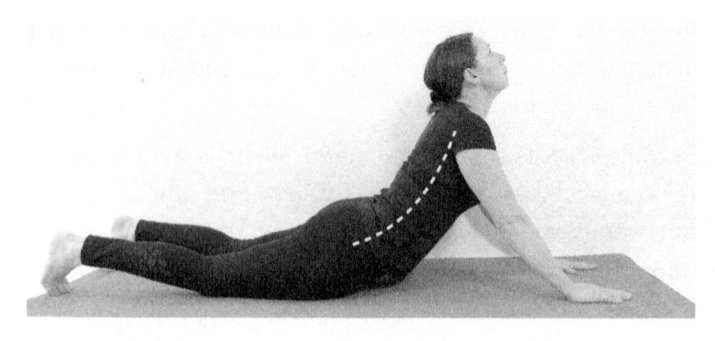

Figure 13.9: The prone extension stretch achieves a high degree of lumbar spine extension.

Extension can also be performed either sitting or standing with these simple actions (**Figure 13.10a,b**).

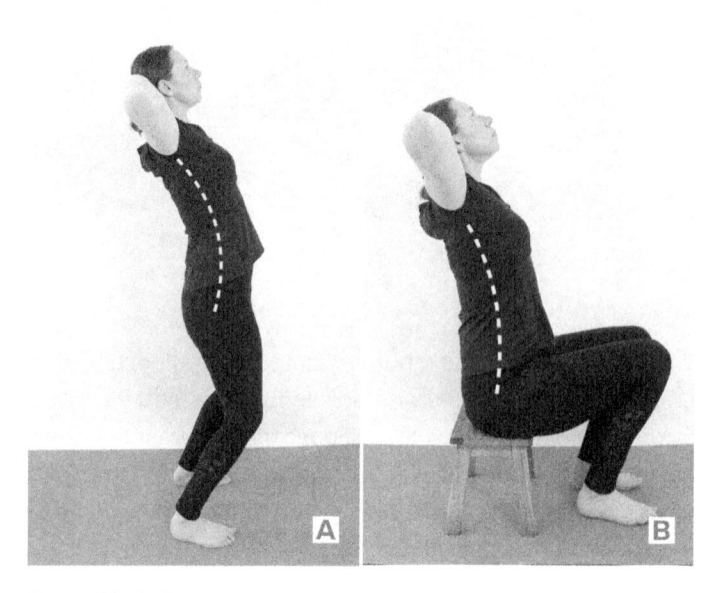

Figure 13.10: Spine extension exercises can be performed in standing (a) and sitting (b).

Overhead reach

For something a little more advanced try this overhead reach (**Figure 13.11**). Start from a supine position, taking your weight through both feet and one hand. Lead with the hand and reach up and over your head while pushing your hips upwards towards the ceiling. You should achieve full extension of your spine and hips and be able to comfortably hold the stretch position for at least 10 seconds. This could be repeated on both sides for a few repetitions.

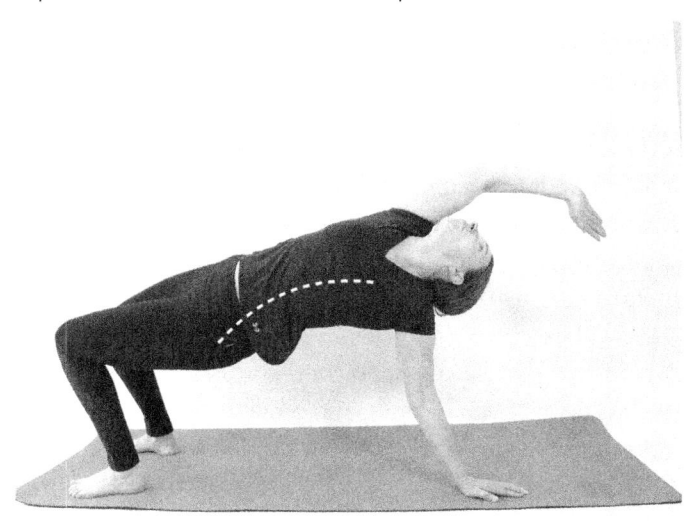

Figure 13.11: The overhead reach can be a fun and challenging spinal extension exercise.

This concludes the extension exercises. In the next section we will focus on strategies to build more resilience.

ADDING LOAD

Many of the exercises we have covered will be useful for both recovery and resilience. They will aid recovery by restoring range of motion and movement confidence and provide opportunities for recalibration of the sensory motor interplay. What is missing from the current approach is load. I use the term load to refer to resistance exercises and weightlifting beyond what can be achieved with simple body weight exercises.

By adding load, we provide a stimulus to build physical strength and resilience; this will increase physical capacity and create a buffer zone or functional reserve of strength. For example, if a client needs to perform childcare duties that involve lifting a toddler, then this may require 75% of the client's maximum strength, leaving them with a 25% reserve. After a strengthening programme, the client may find lifting easier and only require 60% effort to lift the same toddler, leaving them with a 40% reserve. This is an oversimplistic explanation as there are many other factors to consider, but the basic concept is correct. The problem with this example is that toddlers grow quickly!

MOVEMENT VARIABILITY

Another factor to consider is movement variability. Clients undergoing rehabilitation typically perform exercises in specific ways and with good technique, often without much variability. Such precise movement repetition does not reflect the often-awkward movements carried out in normal life. There is an argument for suggesting that this may increase the likelihood of back pain episodes due to the brain receiving unfamiliar sensory feedback from an unusual movement pattern. The completion of varied movement during rehabilitation creates more robust and resilient rehabilitation outcomes.

REPAIR CORTICAL REPRESENTATION

Clients with persistent back pain also have reduced cortical representations in the somatosensory cortex. This means that distortion of sensory input will occur and motor output may be less coordinated, affecting motor control; while not directly linked to pain, there is a correlation between distorted cortical representation and pain.

This alteration has been described as 'smudging' and is allowed to occur due to the brain's ability to modify its neuronal firing patterns. This adaptability is termed cortical plasticity; contrary to what some of our clients believe, the brain can change throughout life and not just in childhood.

PAY ATTENTION WITH PRECISION TRAINING

For positive neuroplastic changes to occur, the brain needs to pay close attention to an input and output. The banal input of a massage or counting thoughtless exercise repetitions does not engage the brain and a significant amount of rehabilitation potential is lost in these non-engaging interventions.

The final component of building resilience is new stimuli. To create a responsive and resilient lower back, you need to develop a responsive and resilient nervous system. We will look at some methods for achieving this.

Adding load: getting started

You can start by just adding some weight to a squat or deadlift. Let us have a look at the deadlift and discuss a few key points:

1. Deconstruct any psychological barriers and explain to your client why they are doing the exercise. Include physical reasons like building strength, reducing the chance of future problems and improving their ability to lift. You could also mention psychological reasons, like improving movement confidence and task confidence. There may be social motivations, like preparing to participate in group exercise or reducing dependency on a partner.

2. Give some movement cues but try to get them started quickly without making an exercise complicated. Aim to build on the positives that your client may be displaying already. Take the opportunity to learn about any movement fears and misconceptions they may have. Common movement myths include: I have to keep my back straight when lifting or I must not let my knees go over my toes when squatting. These are things you can discuss with them. Remember that everybody moves differently and we should aim to embrace this before we look to correct techniques.

3. Once the client is underway, the main thing is that they are doing it and need to do it regularly. At the right time, you could set some efficient exercise parameters using the principles of training but remember to stay focused on understanding and engagement.

We covered exercise parameters in Chapter 8, but to summarise, if the focus is on restoring normal function through neuromuscular activation, then the exercises should be repeated for a set time and could be performed daily at a low intensity (low resistance).

If the focus is strength, then more load will be required and the repetition range will be lower. More rest between sets and between sessions will also be required for adaptation.

MOVEMENT VARIABILITY: GETTING STARTED

The ability to perform a movement in a set way to arrive at the desired position via a narrow movement pathway does not offer much resilience when the uncertainties of a sporting environment or even just normal daily tasks are overlaid. We have already built in some variability during some of the flow exercises as we facilitated motion in all three planes. Here we need to make the tasks more functional and whenever possible add load.

A movement variability drill

Bend down as if preparing to lift the weight, but do not lift it. From the starting phase, move in each plane of motion (**Figure 13.12a–c**):

1. Move forward and back.
2. Move side to side.
3. Twist to each side.

EXERCISE FOR PAIN RELIEF

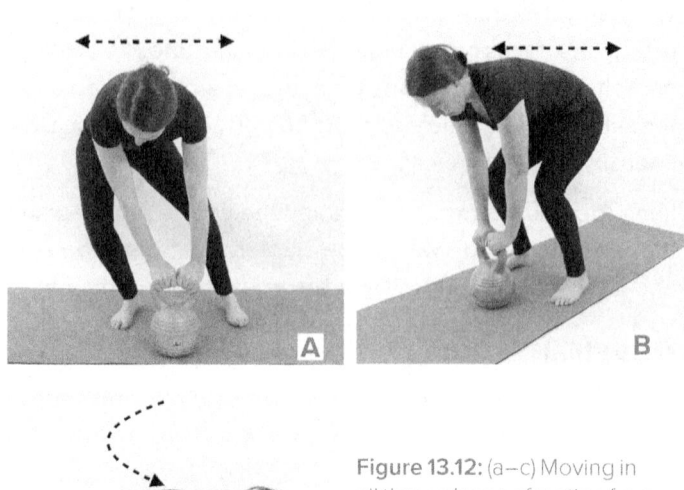

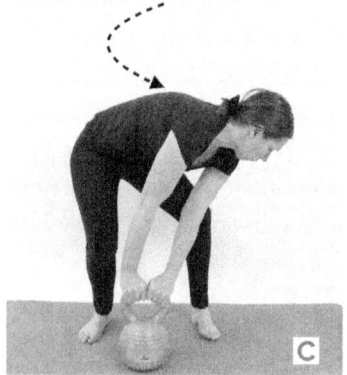

Figure 13.12: (a–c) Moving in all three planes of motion from the lifting start position. Shifting weight laterally to alternate sides from starting position (a). Shifting weight forward and back from starting position (b). Rotating to alternate sides from the starting position (c).

Repeat drill 1, but this time use a light weight to complete a lift for each of the movement variants (**Figure 13.13a–c**).

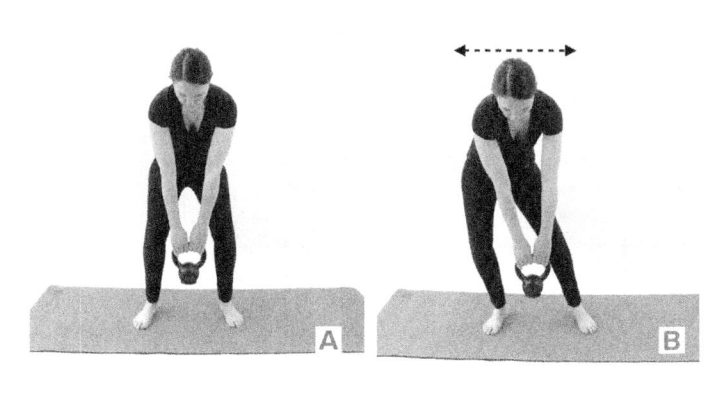

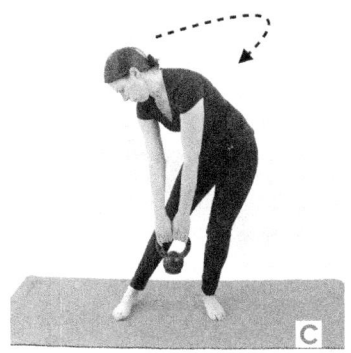

Figure 13.13: (a–c) Lifting from different starting positions to build resilience and confidence. These include neutral (a), lateral weight shifts (b) and rotations (c).

During the variability drills, there is a continued opportunity to assess for movement dysfunctions or behavioural quirks that may help guide other treatment interventions.

PRECISION TRAINING: GETTING STARTED

We previously discussed reduced cortical representation and neuroplasticity along with the need to pay attention to the sensory input and motor output.

Improving sensory input can be achieved with any new stimulus, including massage, tape, foam rolling, cupping and vibration tools. In the clinic, I would justify the use of any of these because the conscious stimulus of an area in combination with consciously controlled movement may help to restore cortical representation.

Motor control may be transiently enhanced by a mechanical stimulus if it is performed just before the exercises, otherwise the nervous system will habituate or return to baseline. The exercises need to have a primary skill component rather than aim to achieve repetitions or time.

We can use many of the exercises we have already used, from the supine pelvic tilt to the lunge twist, with increased focus on the quality of the movement, using a mirror for instant feedback and stopping if movement quality diminishes rather than when muscular fatigue occurs.

Here is a pelvic tilt, self-massage roller drill (Figure 13.14). Sit with a firm core roller on the lumbar spine, then lift your lower back to the top of the roller. Slowly roll down the roller while contracting your abdominals to posteriorly tilt the pelvis. With each motion, you can change the angle to target the lumbar erectors. This drill would couple well with the squat flexion sunrise exercise (**Figure 13.14**).

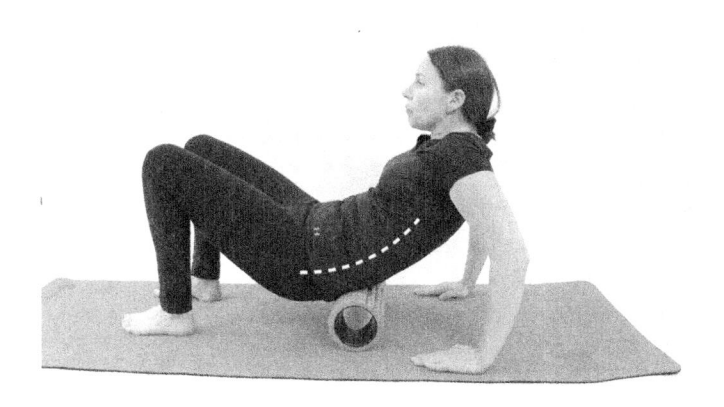

Figure 13.14: A foam roller can be used to massage and exercise the lower back and abdominal muscles.

CONCLUSION

After ruling out any serious pathology, there are many different back pain management approaches; within each approach, there are many exercise options. This chapter has presented concepts, tools and ideas for managing your clients. As always, the challenge is to choose or find the things that are most compatible with each individual client. This chapter aimed to raise awareness of the lack of specificity for back pain rehabilitation and the need to provide exercises with meaning rather than repetition instructions. We discussed how some clients may need more help than others. Many clients suffering an episode of back pain will go through recovery stages where their rehabilitation needs will change. Of the many exercise options available, the aims should stretch beyond simple strength gains to include the restoration of confident and robust movement. In light of the research and modern approaches to lower back pain management, it is important to recognise that lower back pain remains a significant clinical challenge and you can only do your best for your clients.

REFERENCES

Coulombe BJ, Games KE, Neil ER, Eberman LE (2017). Core stability exercise versus general exercise for chronic low back pain. *J Athl Train* 52:71–72.

Keele University. STarT Back Screening Tool. Available at http://www.keele.ac.uk/sbst/ (accessed 19 June 2023).

Malfliet A, Ickmans K, Huysmans E, et al. (2019). Best evidence rehabilitation for chronic pain part 3: low back pain. *J Clin Med* 8:1063.

Norris CM (2019). Back rehabilitation – the 3R's approach. *J Bodyw Mov Ther* 24:289–299.

Steiger F, Wirth B, de Bruin ED, Mannion AF (2011). Is a positive clinical outcome after exercise therapy for chronic non-specific low back pain contingent upon a corresponding improvement in the targeted aspect(s) of performance? A systematic review. *Eur Spine J* 21:575–598.

Vanti C, Andreatta S, Borghi S, et al. (2019). The effectiveness of walking versus exercise on pain and function in chronic low back pain: a systematic review and meta-analysis of randomized trials. *Disabil Rehabil* 41:622–632.

Wand BM, O'Connell NE (2008). Chronic non-specific low back pain – sub-groups or a single mechanism? *BMC Musculoskelet Disord* 9:11.

Wang X-Q, Zheng J-J, Yu Z-W, et al. (2012). A meta-analysis of core stability exercise versus general exercise for chronic low back pain. *PLoS ONE* 7:e52082.

DANIEL LAWRENCE

Lumbar Spine Assessment Videos

Lumbar Spine Treatment Videos

Spinal Education Videos

CHAPTER 14

EXERCISE FOR SHOULDER PAIN

INTRODUCTION

We have arrived at the shoulder joint complex, a complex system of interrelated joints. However, does our exercise approach need to be complicated? Perhaps not!

Let's take a look at some common shoulder problems, research and exercise options. Of the many non-traumatic pathologies that can occur at the shoulder, it is possible to categorise them into three typical presentations as follows.

Shoulder pain syndrome

This has most commonly been called impingement or subacromial impingement. It is also referred to as rotator cuff tendinopathy, but does the terminology matter? Will it change the client's treatment or outcome? We will return to this question later in this chapter. As we know, in health care words really matter; in the case of impingement, we will investigate why.

The stiff shoulder

The stiff shoulder is characterised by a lack of available passive motion. It may be caused by frozen shoulder or glenohumeral contracture syndrome. Shoulders are often stiff after surgery, including surgery for breast cancer. Joint degeneration or prolonged disuse can also lead to a stiff shoulder.

The unstable shoulder

Shoulder instability is a common cause of shoulder pain. Instability can occur after dislocation or because of an existing congenital issue.

The exercise approach for all three shoulder dysfunction categories will be based on the following concepts:

1. Exercises will be limited to a total of 1–3 different exercises.
2. If three exercises are prescribed, they will consist of one primary exercise and two secondary exercises.
3. The primary exercise should be taught with an optional progression and regression to help the client self-manage symptom fluctuations.
4. Advise the client to keep an exercise diary to identify longer-term patterns and reduce unwanted attention on acute pain fluctuations.

EXERCISE FOR SHOULDER PAIN SYNDROME

I consider a study by British physiotherapist and researcher Dr Chris Littlewood (Littlewood et al., 2016) as one of the most groundbreaking shoulder physical therapy studies of recent years. For decades clinicians have been teaching shoulder exercises for common shoulder pain presentations, advancing exercise knowledge, developing increasingly complex rehabilitation programmes and prescribing specific exercises based on a suspected structural pathology. On the receiving end of these clinical exercise plans, clients are often overwhelmed by the complexity or amount of exercises and unfortunately often underwhelmed by the results of their exercise efforts. You may have experienced this in your own clinic; despite your best efforts and the client's diligent exercise completion, their shoulder still hurts!

The solution may be to dial back the exercises, potentially just focusing on one exercise, while rebalancing exercise with strategies to understand and accept a degree of shoulder pain with exercise and activity. The client's willingness to exercise in the presence of some pain is important especially as it may take several weeks to achieve some meaningful pain relief. As a guide, shoulder pain during exercise should be acceptable to the client and return back to baseline after exercise completion. A sustained post-exercise flare-up of pain would require an adjustment to the exercise plan.

THE EXERCISE

The exercise should target the most symptomatic movement of the shoulder and be taught with progressions and regressions that afford the client the ability to self-manage their exercise programme in response to natural symptom fluctuations. As mentioned, pain is acceptable if it does not worsen after stopping the exercise. Although acceptable, pain is not necessary and if you can help the client to find an exercise or way of performing it that is more comfortable, this will lead to an increased likelihood of the client adhering to the exercise. I often tell my clients that although pain is acceptable during shoulder exercises, it is not necessary, and they should not hesitate to adjust their exercises to increase comfort. This advice sits in-between the common advice to 'stop if it hurts' or 'no pain, no gain', both unhelpfully polarised options that fail to guide clients aiming to achieve pain relief from exercise.

The single exercise could be an isometric or dynamic abduction (**Figure 14.1**), lateral rotation (**Figure 14.2**) or flexion (**Figure 14.3**). The specific intervention in the study by Littlewood et al. (2016) was one of these exercises for 3 sets of 10–15 repetitions twice per day.

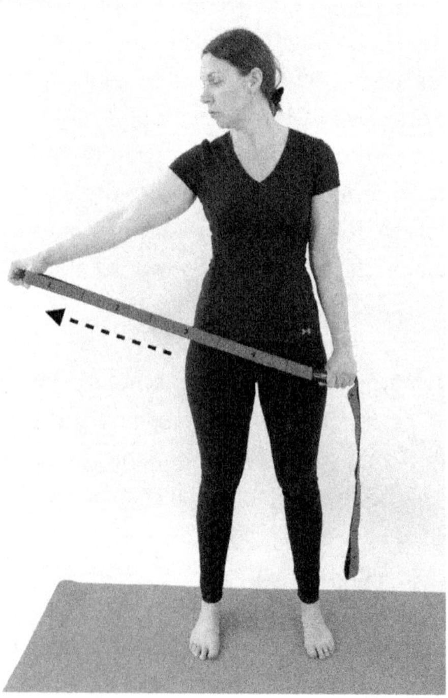

Figure 14.1: The dynamic abduction exercise can be performed isometrically or dynamically.

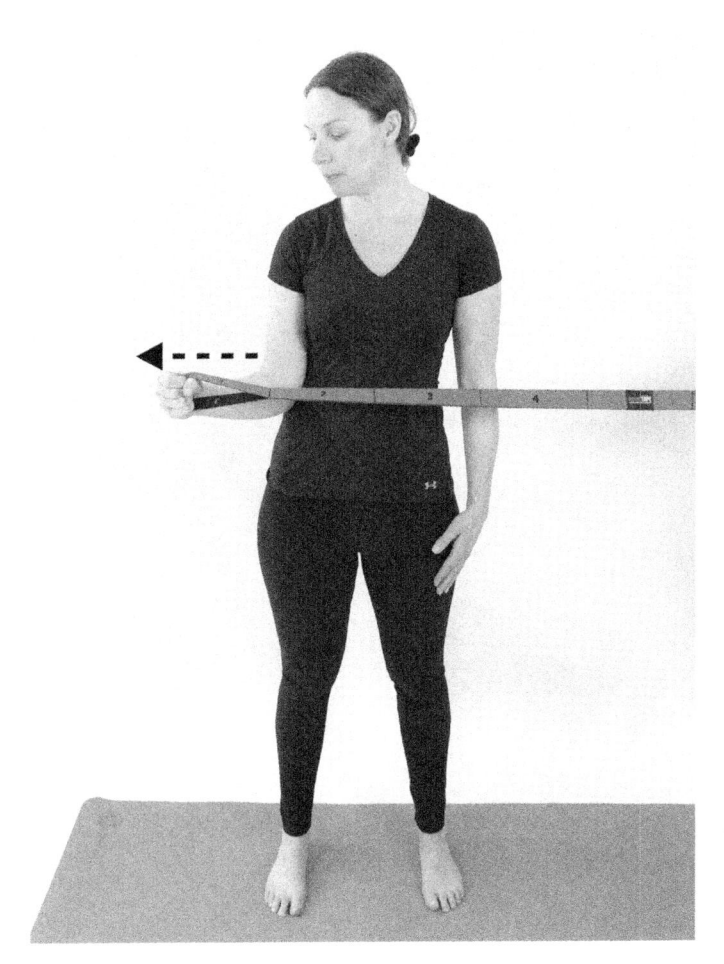

Figure 14.2: The lateral rotation exercise is a simple shoulder exercise that many people are familiar with.

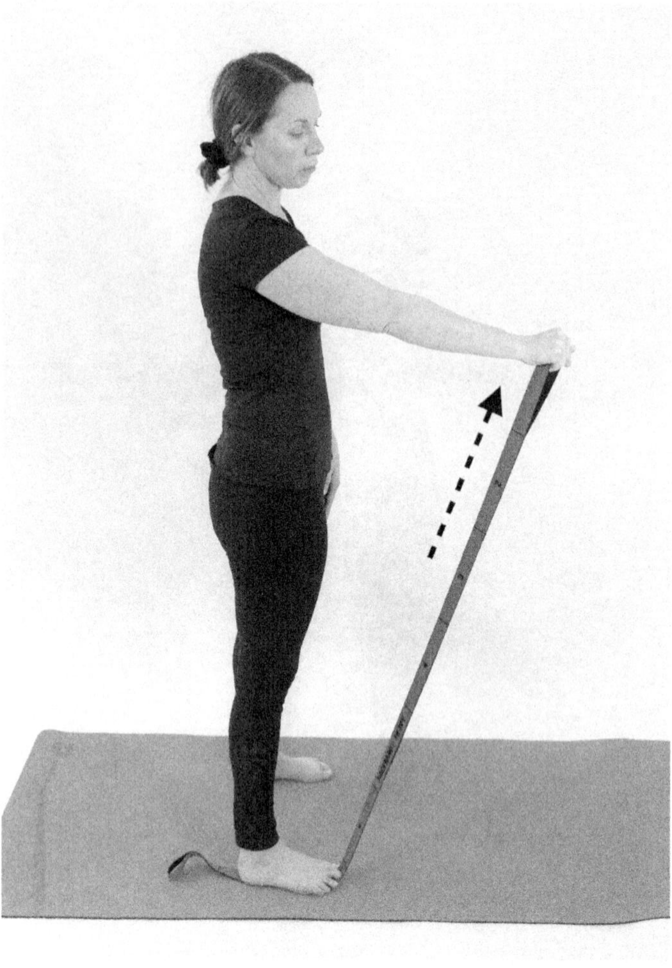

Figure 14.3: Shoulder flexion is a simple shoulder exercise option.

If you believe that doing 3 sets of 10–15 repetitions twice a day is not an effective exercise plan and goes against exercise principles, you might be overlooking the main goal here. While it may not be the best plan for building muscle strength, it is important to note that this study did not focus on improving shoulder strength specifically. Its aim was to enhance overall function where strength is just one aspect among many.

In conclusion, Littlewood and colleagues (2016) demonstrated that a self-management programme based around a single exercise is comparable to usual physiotherapy treatment, saving time, resources and money, and allowing a focus on more cognitive strategies. In the clinic, I have found that clients achieve better outcomes and report higher satisfaction from this simpler style of approach.

I believe that the interaction with the client is also an opportunity to improve regional function and that offering just one isolated exercise for one joint on one side of the body is potentially a missed opportunity. In my experience, I like to add another couple of general regional functional exercises. My two favourites are:

- Banded row with thoracic flexion and extension (**Figure 14.4**). This exercise promotes healthy scapulothoracic function and actively mobilises the thoracic spine.

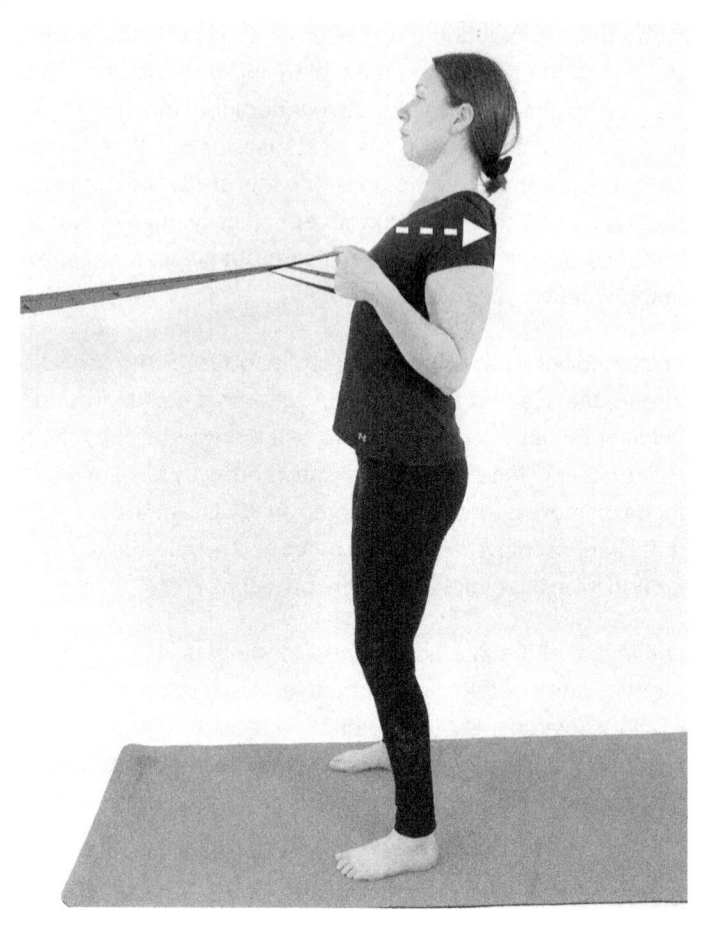

Figure 14.4: The banded row with thoracic flexion and extension.

- Banded push with thoracic extension to flexion (**Figure 14.5**). This is the opposite of the first exercise and again it gets many muscles and joints moving in this region, including the serratus anterior.

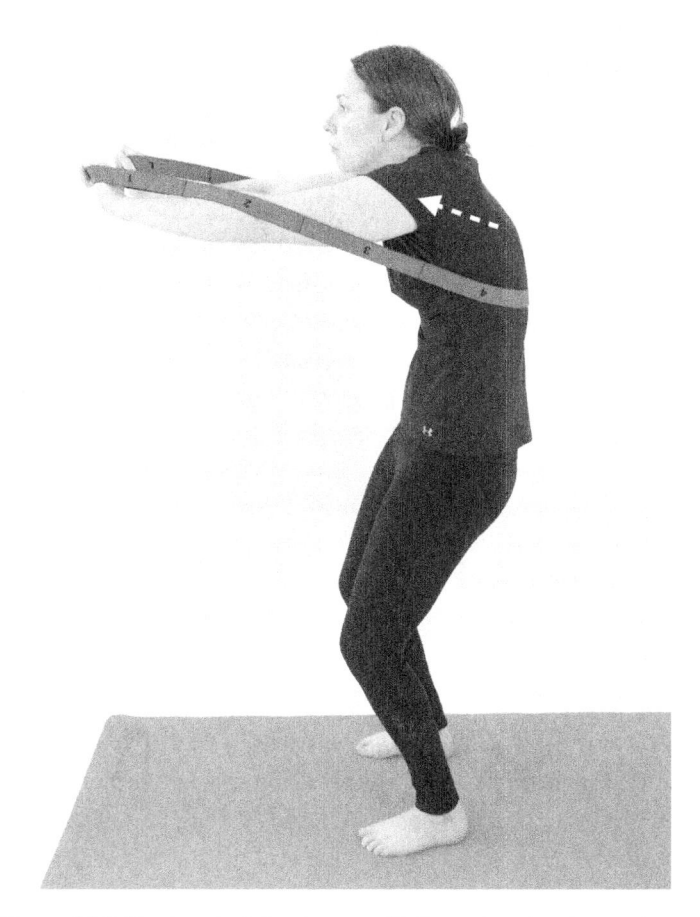

Figure 14.5: The banded chest press with thoracic extension and flexion.

EXERCISE FOR THE STIFF SHOULDER

As mentioned, a stiff shoulder could be caused by multiple factors, including a frozen shoulder, post-fracture, surgical procedures, general disuse and joint changes.

I recommend using these three exercise principles to improve range of motion:

1. Target the joint end ranges. Mainly forward flexion (elevation) and external rotation.
2. Manipulate the stretch reflex by contracting and relaxing muscles at or towards their current end ranges.
3. Use eccentric contractions that move into the joint end ranges.

Based on the fact that forward flexion and external rotation are typically the two most limited movements for a stiff shoulder, we will now go through three exercises for these two motions.

The exercises

Stick stretch

From a standing or kneeling position, firmly grip a stick as high as possible and then slowly lower your body to increase the stretch through the shoulder **(figure 14.6).** From this end-range stretched position, you can reduce the stretch reflex by pushing the stick down into the ground to create a sustained end-range isometric contraction. You can also use eccentric muscle contractions by releasing some tension to move out of the joint's end range. You can push the stick down again followed by a controlled lowering of your body, so you eccentrically lengthen into elevation. This means that you start with an isometric contraction near the end range; then, lowering your body consciously overpowers the isometric contraction so that an eccentric lengthening contraction occurs into the end range. This promotes sarcomerogenesis, which is the formation and development of new muscle fibres, also termed sarcomeres. This does not occur in just one session, so any immediate gains are likely to be from reductions in stretch reflex sensitivity.

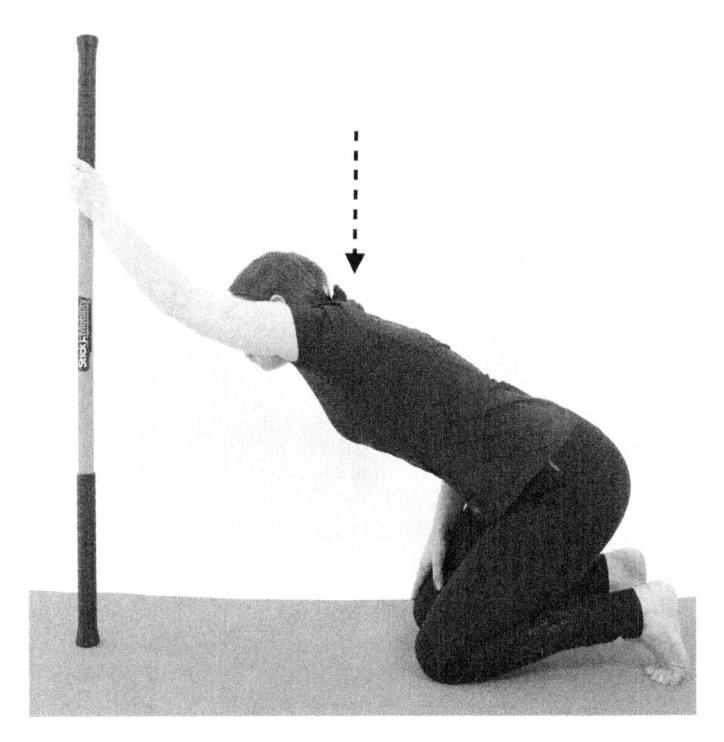

Figure 14.6: The stick stretch can be performed at home with a mop or broom handle.

Supine dumbbell elevation

From a supine position, hold a weight above your head and then eccentrically lower the weight above your head as far as possible, hold for a few seconds and then return to the start position (**Figure 14.7**). Once the client has mastered this simple motion, progress the exercise with an isometric contraction at the end of the range and then nudge further into the elevation, or work on eccentrically lowering into the end range repeatedly. In the clinic, I find that the contract–relax technique is the most effective at achieving increased joint range with this exercise.

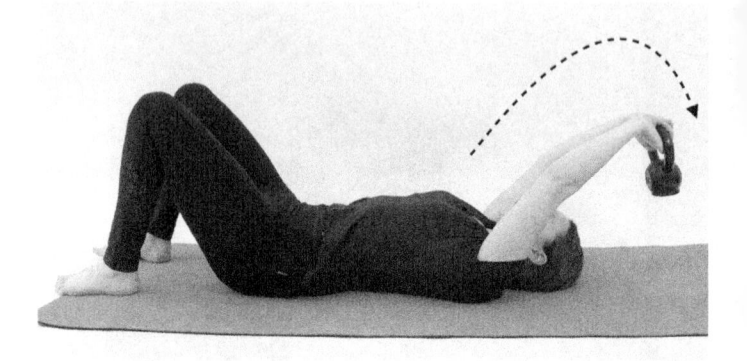

Figure 14.7: The supine dumbbell elevation exercise can help to increase joint range.

ASSISTED OR RESISTED EXTERNAL ROTATION

A stick can be used to facilitate an effective external rotation drill. Bend the elbows and hold the stick in front of you, then actively externally rotate the shoulder as far as possible. The stick can then be used to drive the shoulder further into external rotation using the other arm to provide the force (**Figure 14.8**). I find it most effective to take the shoulder to the end of the tolerable range then push back isometrically towards internal rotation for a few seconds, followed by an assisted external rotation. This should be repeated 1–3 times.

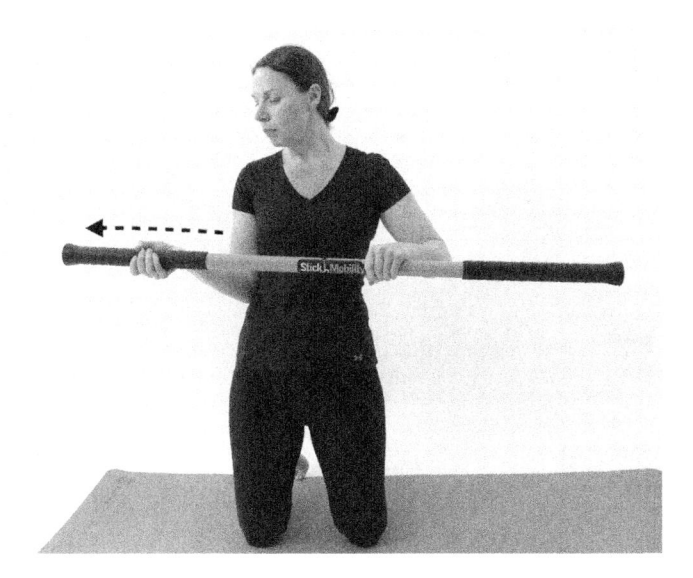

Figure 14.8: A stick can be used to perform the external rotation exercise.

I have had success with these specific exercises, but I am aware that there are similar alternatives. I would strongly suggest that whatever techniques you use, you should aim to target end-ranges, manipulate the stretch reflex and use eccentric contractions.

THE UNSTABLE SHOULDER

An unstable shoulder commonly presents as highly mobile, often painful and with specific instability and apprehension signs.

Regular activation of the rotator cuff within the mid-range will help to increase muscle tone and the feeling of joint support while avoiding promoting laxity into the end ranges. External and internal rotation can be performed with a focus on neuromuscular activation (**Table 14.1**). Progression can then be achieved by adding progressive abduction and resistance.

Table 14.1: Neuromuscular activation guidelines (these are the suggested exercise parameters for neuromuscular activation)

GUIDELINE	DESCRIPTION
Load	Low – 30% + 1RM or less
Repetitions	30–60 seconds
Sets	1–5
Rest	60 seconds
Weekly sessions	5–7 days
Speed	Moderate-to-slow or isometric
Fatigue	Low-to-moderate, not to failure

The exercises

With the arm by the side of the body and elbow bent to 90 degrees, choose whether to perform external **(Figure 14.9)** or internal rotation (**Figure 14.10**). Perform each exercise in a controlled manner and, as mentioned initially, avoid end-range positions. This exercise can be progressed in many ways, including by adding progressive levels of abduction before performing the external rotation (**Figure 14.11**).

Standing snow angels are a more advanced stability exercise option (**Figure 14.12**). To perform this exercise, pull two resistance bands into external glenohumeral joint rotation bilaterally and then abduct your shoulders while maintaining the external rotation. In case you were wondering, if you lie in the snow and perform this action, it will leave an angel-shaped imprint.

So that covers the three types of shoulder dysfunction. Before we move on up to the neck in the next chapter, I want to present one more study that relates to the shoulder, the neck and exercise for pain relief in general.

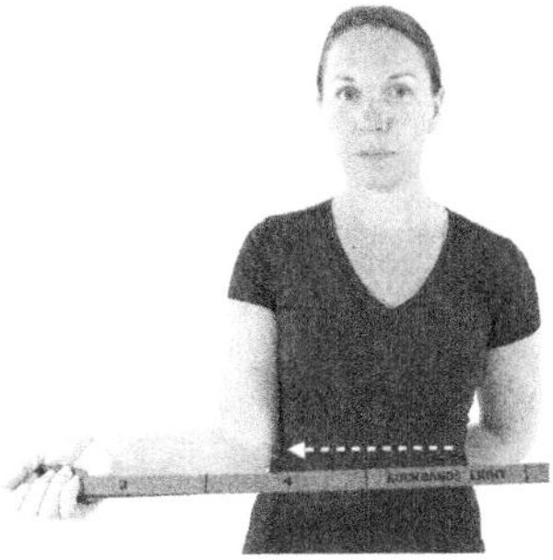

Figure 14.9: Glenohumeral external rotation.

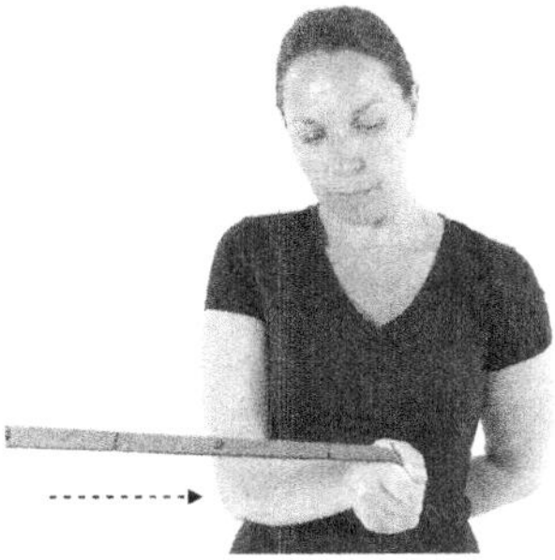

Figure 14.10: Glenohumeral internal rotation.

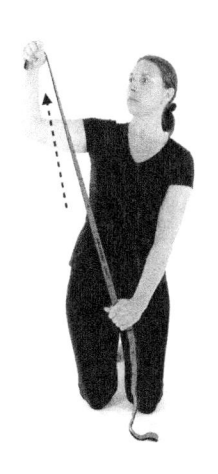

Figure 14.11: External rotation in abduction.

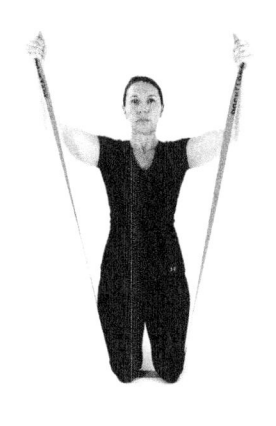

Figure 14.12: Standing snow angel exercise.

RESEARCH REVIEW

A study by Anderson and colleagues (2011) set out to determine the effectiveness of just 2 minutes of daily neck and shoulder exercise using an elastic tube for resistance. The authors measured to see if this small amount of exercise would be sufficient to reduce reported pain and tenderness; they also measured abduction shoulder strength.

They studied a total of 174 patients with shoulder and neck pain over a 10-week period to assess their response to 1 of 3 interventions. One group only received information on general health. One group did 12 minutes of shoulder and neck exercises 5 days a week and one group did 2 minutes of shoulder and neck exercises 5 days a week.

Both exercise groups reported superior results to the non-exercise group, but the key finding was that even the 2-minute exercise group reported significant pain reduction and demonstrated strength increases closely matched to the 12-minute group with no discernible difference identified.

Two key messages come out of this study. First, just doing a little bit of targeted exercise can make a significant difference. In this study, as little as 2 minutes made a difference. You have to wonder what the outcome would have been if they had groups doing as little as 1 minute or 30 seconds. How little exercise can you get away with?

Second, doing exercise daily creates an adherence-promoting routine. Sometimes, if a patient is required to engage in strengthening just 2–3 times a week, the likelihood of them missing a session and falling out of a routine is potentially increased rather than decreased. This may be because a ritualistic pattern is more likely to emerge from repeating a daily task.

IS 'IMPINGEMENT' A NOCEBO WORD?

The term impingement has been used as a diagnosis for glenohumeral joint pain for decades. First described in 1972 by Dr Charles Neer, it is still the most common shoulder diagnosis to this day. However, it is a misdiagnosis and has been described as a nocebo term due to its suggestion that a structural squashing of the tendon under the acromion every time the patient attempts to lift their arm is responsible for the pain. This often makes patients feel more pain and move less; they also show reduced willingness to complete exercise rehabilitation, thus increasing the propensity for surgery. Research showed that cuff tendon tears occur not between the acromion and the tendon; instead, they most frequently occur between the humeral head and the tendon (Payne et al., 1997). In terms of surgery, findings from a large multicentre surgical study reported that subacromial decompression surgery has no additional benefit over placebo (sham) surgery (Beard et al., 2018).

CONCLUSION

Bringing this chapter together helped me to become more effective at treating shoulder pain; I hope it offers you the same road to success. I think one of the key concepts is that once you select the exercises that target the dysfunctions, you then need to help the client understand why you have prescribed these exercises and what they can expect to experience both during and after the exercises. I do not believe that there is such a thing as the best shoulder exercise, that is, unless the client reports it as such.

REFERENCES

Andersen LL, Saervoll CA, Mortensen OS, et al. (2011). Effectiveness of small daily amounts of progressive resistance training for frequent neck/shoulder pain: randomised controlled trial. *Pain* 152:440–446.

Beard DJ, Rees JL, Cook JA, et al. (2018). Arthroscopic subacromial decompression for subacromial shoulder pain (CSAW): a multicentre, pragmatic, parallel group, placebo-controlled, three-group, randomised surgical trial. *Lancet* 391:329–338.

Littlewood C, Bateman M, Brown K, et al. (2016). A self-managed single exercise programme versus usual physiotherapy treatment for rotator cuff tendinopathy: a randomised controlled trial (the SELF study). *Clin Rehabil* 30:686–696.

Payne LZ, Altchek DW, Craig EV, Warren RF (1997). Arthroscopic treatment of partial rotator cuff tears in young athletes. A preliminary report. *Am J Sports Med* 25:299–305.

Shoulder Assessment Videos   Shoulder Treatment Videos

CHAPTER 15

EXERCISE FOR NECK PAIN

INTRODUCTION

Personally, I have always found neck pain more difficult to manage than thoracic or lumbar spine pain. Structurally, the cervical spine is not as robust as the lumbar spine and overall clients have less tolerance for movement interventions. The neck also serves the senses in a way that no other part of the body does. That is to say, it moves the head in response to visual, auditory and other stimuli. Some accessory muscles of breathing are also cervical muscles; therefore, breathing pattern disorders may have an influence on neck function. Neck tension has a close association with stress, and psychological factors can be more influential on the recovery from an acute bout of non-traumatic neck pain than physical factors (Wirth et al., 2016). If your clinical experiences are anything like mine, you will have struggled to offer your clients credible and helpful neck pain exercises. You may have prescribed neck strengthening exercises, for which there is good evidence and justification, but they are often awkward to perform and impractical to do. I find adherence is low and clients report them being uncomfortable; it also messes up their hair if they start wrapping elastic exercise bands around their head!

In this chapter, I present some simple and convenient neck exercise strategies that should reduce neck pain. I have found these exact same exercises successful in the clinic and they each have a theoretical justification for their inclusion in this chapter. As always, the main aim is to reduce pain. If a more specific strengthening programme is required, I would advise seeking a more strength-and-conditioning-based programme.

A full assessment is recommended before beginning neck exercises. In the absence of any serious symptoms, the exercises outlined in this chapter can be trialled for neck pain of different levels of severity. Because neck pain often has a strong cognitive and behavioural component, you may need to refer back to Chapter 6 to help tackle non-physical barriers. For example, a specific subgroup of clients with a whiplash-associated disorder often present a complex biopsychosocial challenge. That is to say, they are more difficult to treat.

EXERCISE CATEGORIES

The exercises presented in this chapter can be categorised as follows:

- Functional movement activities.
- Specific strengthening and motor control tasks.
- Breathing pattern retraining.

FUNCTIONAL MOVEMENT ACTIVITIES

As mentioned, the neck serves our senses, including vision. Research has shown that vision-oriented tasks can be used to rehabilitate the neck. There is a close working relationship between vision and the neck muscles that keeps our gaze stable when the head and neck moves, this occurs naturally when we walk and perform other daily tasks. You can try a gaze stability test now as you read this paragraph. Focus on this WORD and then move your head side to side and up and down while maintaining a stable gaze on the word. The movement of your head was voluntary but the countermovement of your eyes was automatic thanks to a clever reflex.

This reflex is called the cervico-ocular reflex (COR). Neck pain can cause dizziness and balance issues due to sensory disruption to the COR (de Vries et al., 2016; Ischebeck et al., 2018). The inner ear also has a vestibulo-ocular reflex that helps to keep our body and vision stable.

Returning back to vision and neck pain, virtual reality studies have identified that by manipulating the visual perception of rotation, it is possible to increase or decrease the available range of motion in individuals with neck pain (Chen et al., 2017; Harvie et al., 2015). The method used by Harvie and colleagues (2015) was to use visual virtual reality technology that detected neck rotation and then displayed the rotation visually to the participants through the virtual reality headset. The clever part was the ability of that visual representation to display an increased or decreased rotation, leading participants to feel that they had rotated further or not as far as they had physically in real life. When participants were shown images of an increased rotation, they physically rotated less. When they were shown a reduced rotation image, they rotated further. The point at which they reported pain and the available range of active motion were directly influenced by the sensory information from the eyes. So, not only can neck pain cause visual issues, but vision-oriented tasks can be used to rehabilitate the neck. This is a very important fact to remember and will serve you well when dealing with clients with neck pain.

At the time of writing, it was possible but not practical to use virtual reality headsets for home exercises. It may soon be a reality that most people will have a virtual reality headset and an augmented reality neck pain app will provide a pragmatic way of using the research we have just been discussing.

I recommend letting visual stimuli lead your functional rehabilitation exercises. This allows the neck to naturally serve the senses; it gives the neck a reason to move and a goal-oriented outcome. A visual stimulus also offers a distraction and may help to reduce pain hypervigilance, which is all too common with a typical range of motion exercise.

Perhaps you could explain it to clients in this way. Turning the head while expecting some pain is not a very enticing exercise, but turning the head for a pleasant stimulus or one of interest is more motivating, functional and more natural.

Here are three vision-led functional exercises that are generally well accepted by patients:

1. Torso rotation (**Figure 15.1**). The neck rotates when we turn our head, obviously, but it also rotates if we keep the head still and rotate the body; it is the same movement but the context is different and the visual field does not change.

Because you are not producing a rotational visual input, a more pain-free range may be achieved. If possible, I like to do this exercise on a rotating chair. If this is not an option, then it can be done from a normal chair or standing. This task is a little better if you keep your head facing an object and your gaze is fixed on something pleasant or interesting. I recommend a nice picture on the wall of your clinic to help with your neck rehabilitation sessions.

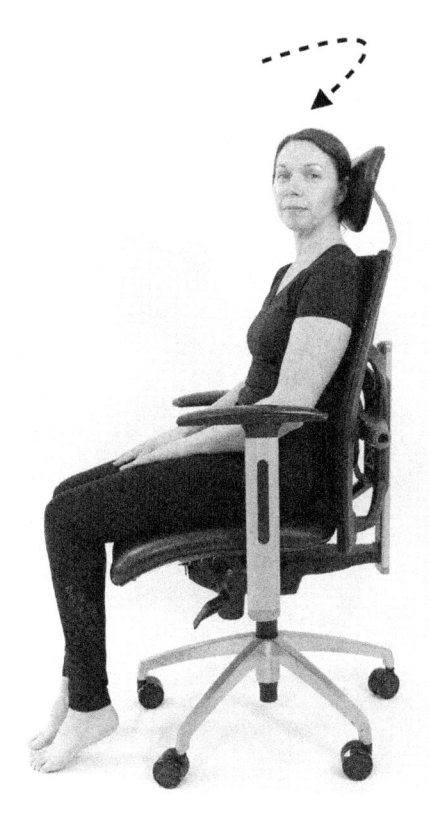

Figure 15.1: The torso rotation exercise is a simple neck rehabilitation exercise.

EXERCISE FOR PAIN RELIEF

2. Window shopping. The aim is to rotate the head in response to a stimulus just as if you were walking past a shop window (**Figure 15.2**). Walk past something like a plant, picture or window and turn your head as you walk past it, fixing your gaze for as long as possible. It is basically neck rotation but in a functional context. It is easy for clients to do this in the house or garden (if they have one).

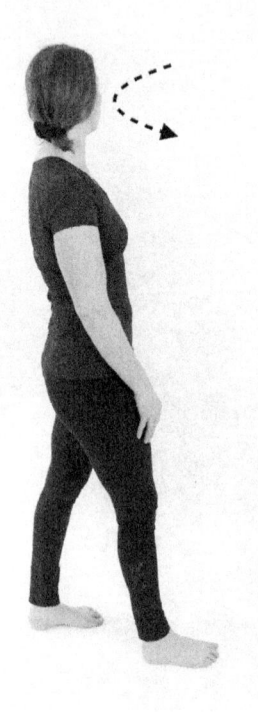

Figure 15.2: The window shopping exercise is another torso rotation exercise option.

3. Gaze stability (**Figure 15.3**). Here we can work on the reflexes between the neck muscles, the ocular muscles and the vestibular system. Instruct your client to fix their gaze on a picture or anything that is not moving and then move the head; first, try rotations then flexions and extensions and then any direction while maintaining a stable gaze on the target.

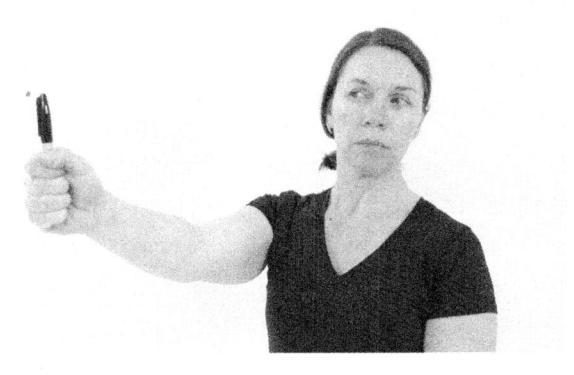

Figure 15.3: The gaze stability exercise

STRENGTHENING AND MOTOR CONTROL EXERCISES

Strengthening exercises have been shown to correlate with reduced neck pain; weakening of the cervical musculature has been reported in individuals with neck pain. More specifically, reductions in maximal voluntary contraction, fibre type changes and fatty infiltration can occur. Engaging in muscle strengthening exercises around the neck is a popular and evidence-based approach to pain management. However, we often come up against a barrier; clients often hold the belief that the neck is a delicate structure and feel tension

EXERCISE FOR PAIN RELIEF

and pain around their neck. They are told to relax, take it easy and avoid straining their neck.

When a well-informed therapist then suggests resistance training for their neck, it can create mixed messages with clients remaining concerned that exercise may strain their neck or increase their tension further. Once again, you may need to use some strategies from Chapter 6 of the book to build your clients' confidence.

For this chapter, the challenge was to present the most effective neck exercises that have the highest client compliance. Here are two exercises that I often teach my clients:

1. Cervico-occipital flexion (**Figure 15.4**). There are many justifications for this exercise; it targets the deep cervical flexors and if done correctly reduces habitual activation of the sternocleidomastoid. The suboccipital region also responds to this exercise, which may reduce upper cervical dysfunction and cervicogenic headaches. The exercise also feels therapeutic because it requires submaximal muscle contraction and is easy to perform correctly.

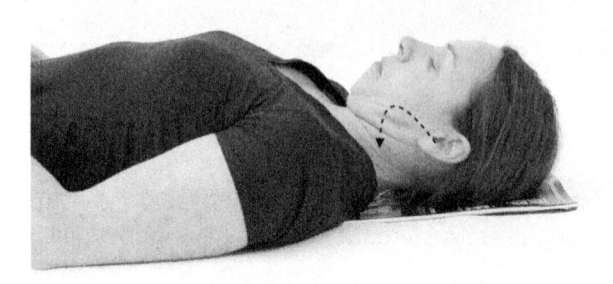

Figure 15.4: Cervico-occipital flexion can be performed while supine. A magazine will provide a low-friction surface.

2. Shoulder shrugs (**Figure 15.5**) take advantage of the fact that many neck muscles also serve as elevators of the shoulder girdle. By engaging these muscles with shoulder shrug exercises, it is possible to add considerable resistance without feeling the strain on the neck.

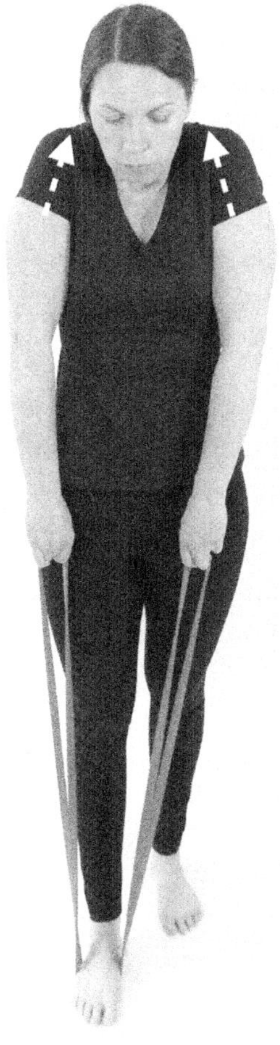

Figure 15.5: The shoulder shrug exercise.

After these exercises, if the client feels a benefit, it would then be an option to include some more vigorous neck-specific loading, if necessary. With a neck that is unresponsive to treatment, a strengthening stimulus may provide the missing ingredient that is required for rehabilitation progress.

BREATHING PATTERN RETRAINING

It is typical for an individual with neck pain to report tension and tenderness across their upper shoulders and for this feeling to be commonly exacerbated by stress. Breathing pattern disorders may help to explain the link between stress and neck pain. As stated previously, psychosocial factors can be more influential on recovery from non-traumatic neck pain than physical factors (Wirth et al., 2016).

Let us consider this potential mechanism: anxiety triggers the release of adrenaline which elevates the heart and breathing rates. This is obvious with a traumatic event like falling over or being startled, but even a small boost of adrenaline can occur from something minor like a smartphone notification.

An increased breathing rate is a natural response to a stimulus, but with repeated increases in anxiety or a maintained state of anxiety, a hyperventilation pattern can occur that alters muscle tone and respiratory patterns. Clients often show signs of reduced diaphragmatic breathing and increased activity in the accessory muscles of breathing, many of which have cervical attachments.

Hyperventilation can also cause hypocapnia, which is a reduction in carbon dioxide levels in the blood; this alters blood chemistry and can cause a myriad of medically unexplained symptoms like disorientation, brain fog and paraesthesia. Perhaps somewhat paradoxically, these symptoms can also cause anxiety, having been caused by anxiety in the first instance.

Breathing pattern assessment, awareness and retraining is a pragmatic way to reduce anxiety, stress and tension. It may provide a credible self-management strategy for reducing a client's neck pain.

BREATHING PATTERN RETRAINING

It is possible that the client may not have any issues with their breathing pattern. This next exercise (**Figure 15.6**) can be used for breathing pattern assessment and re-education; if no breathing pattern re-education is necessary, it can still serve as a simple relaxation exercise that may help to reduce pain and anxiety.

Sitting in a chair, ask your client to place one hand over their upper abdomen and one hand over their chest. The placement of the hands will indicate the amount of expansion occurring at the abdomen and chest during inhalation. The client should be instructed to breath normally and avoid any forced deeper inhalation. Relaxed breathing should occur through the nose, be quiet and consist of about 12–16 breaths per minute.

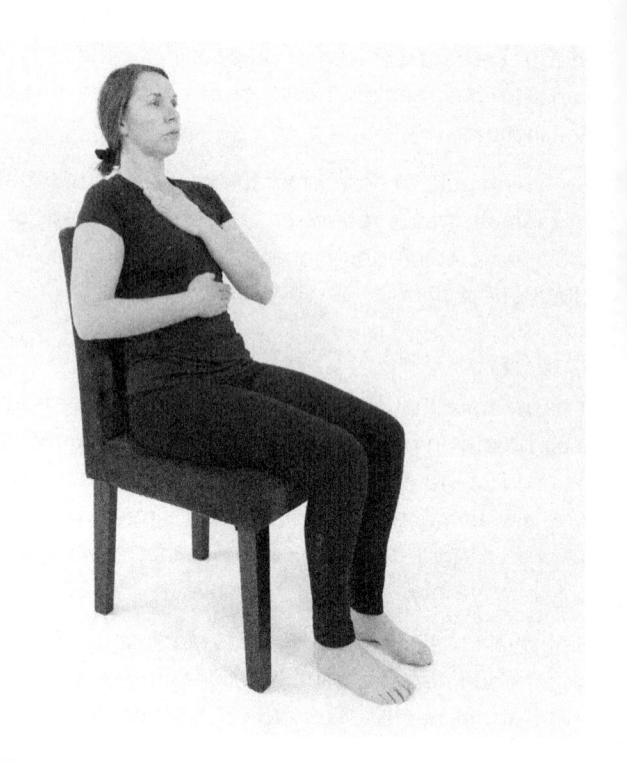

Figure 15.6: Breathing pattern retraining with hand placement over the upper abdomen and chest to self-assess diaphragm and upper chest expansion.

It is possible to consciously change the naturally unconscious movement pattern of breathing. This can be achieved by first being aware of the current breathing pattern and then having some simple strategies to retrain the pattern if necessary. It is often as simple as educating the client about their current breathing pattern and then facilitating some changes to enhance the contribution of the diaphragm. For example, the client can be instructed to slow the out breath and then use their lower hand to feel for a relaxed abdominal expansion during inhalation.

CONCLUSION

When it comes to neck pain, we may be guilty of looking for physical dysfunctions, performing special tests, finding tight muscles and diagnosing stiff joints.

We simply do not spend enough time listening for psychological barriers, understanding client perceptions and appreciating their personal goals. Neck pain is especially sensitive to psychological, biological and social factors.

The neck's close working alliance with the eyes and vestibular system can also be used to enhance rehabilitation outcomes, while breathing pattern disorders provide a treatment bridge between the impact of stress and muscle tension around the neck.

REFERENCES

Chen KB, Sesto ME, Ponto, et al. (2017). Use of virtual reality feedback for patients with chronic neck pain and kinesiophobia. *IEEE Trans Neural Syst Rehabil Eng* 25:1240–1248.

de Vries J, Ischebeck BK, Voogt LP, et al. (2016). Cervico-ocular reflex is increased in people with nonspecific neck pain. *Phys Ther* 96:1190–1195.

Harvie DS, Broecker M, Smith RT, et al. (2015). Bogus visual feedback alters onset of movement–evoked pain in people with neck pain. *Psychol Sci* 26:385–392.

Ischebeck BK, de Vries J, van Wingerden JP, et al. (2018). The influence of cervical movement on eye stabilization reflexes: a randomized trial. *Exp Brain Res* 236:297–304.

Wirth B, Humphreys BK, Peterson C (2016). Importance of psychological factors for the recovery from a first episode of acute non-specific neck pain: a longitudinal observational study. *Chiropr Man Ther* 24:9.

BIBLIOGRAPHY

Rezaei I, Razeghi M, Ebrahimi S, Kayedi S, Rezaeian Zadeh A (2019). A novel virtual reality technique (Cervigame®) compared to conventional proprioceptive training to treat neck pain: a randomized controlled trial. *J Biomed Phys Eng* 9:355–366.

Neck Assessment Videos

Neck Treatment Videos

THE PHYSIO CHANNEL

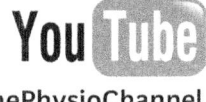

You Tube @ThePhysioChannel

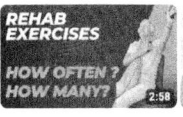

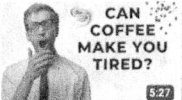

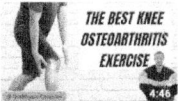

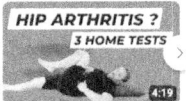

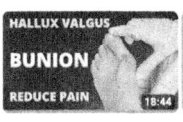

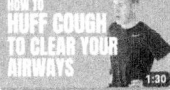

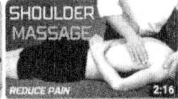

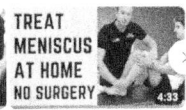

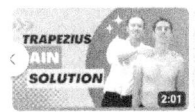

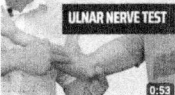

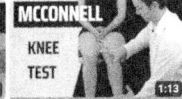

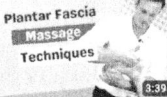

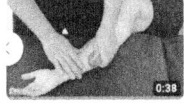

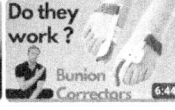

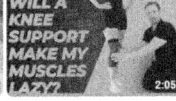

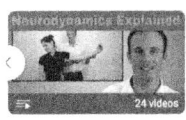

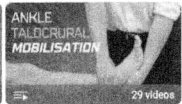

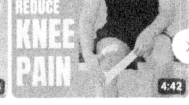

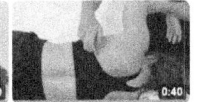

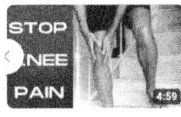

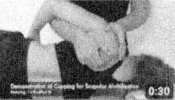

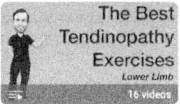

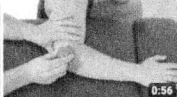

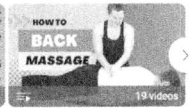

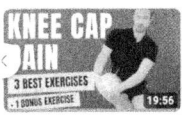

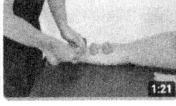

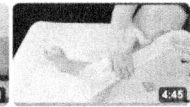

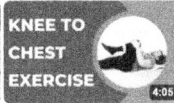

Physical Therapy videos for professionals, students and patients on the YouTube channel.

Also available...

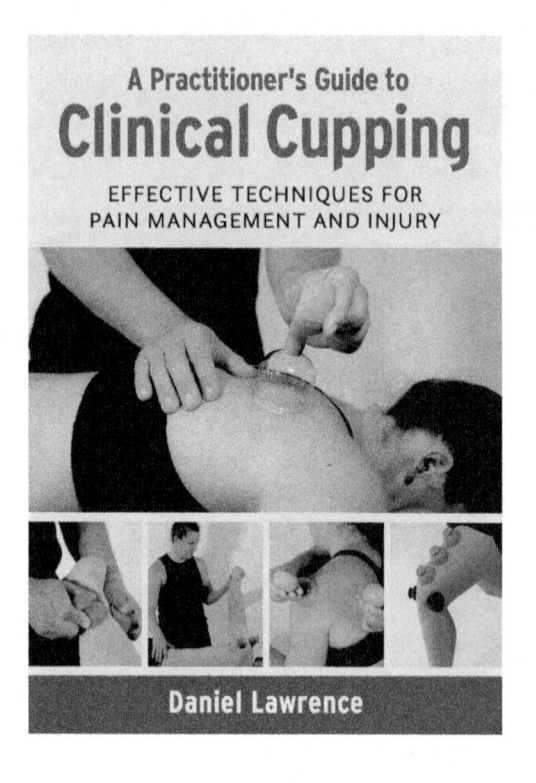

A Practitioner's Guide to
Clinical Cupping
EFFECTIVE TECHNIQUES FOR PAIN MANAGEMENT AND INJURY

Daniel Lawrence

In this highly practical guide, acclaimed physical therapist and international lecturer Daniel Lawrence dispels some of the myths around cupping therapy and shows how it deserves to be viewed as a highly credible and versatile therapeutic tool in modern practice

Also available...

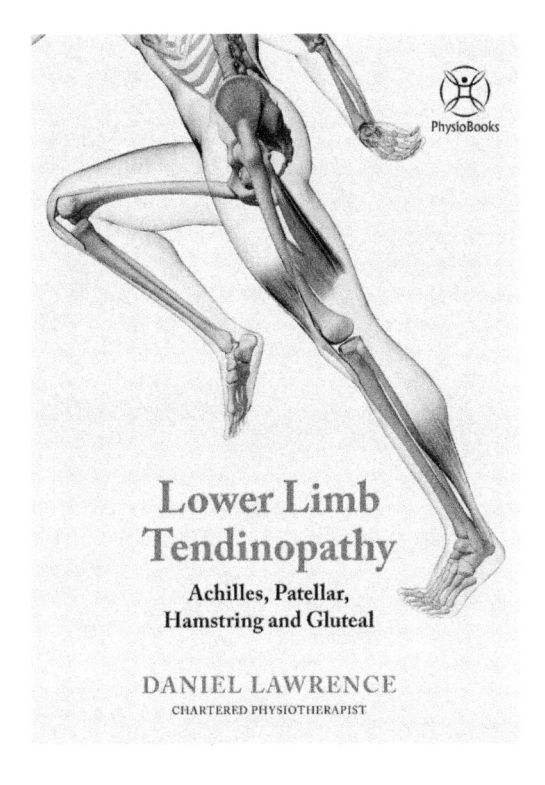

Lower Limb Tendinopathy
Achilles, Patellar, Hamstring and Gluteal

DANIEL LAWRENCE
CHARTERED PHYSIOTHERAPIST

A comprehensive guide for professionals involved in the management of lower limb tendon pain and dysfunction. Extensively researched with over 300 references this book combines evidence with clinical experience to provide informed tendinopathy management strategies. Extensively illustrated with over 200 images and diagrams plus summarised clinical assessment guides and rehabilitation plans.